THE 28-DAY
BLOOD SUGAR
MIRACLE

THE 28-DAY BLOOD SUGAR MIRACLE

Cher Pastore
MS, RD, CDE®

A Revolutionary Diet Plan to Get Your Diabetes Under Control in Less Than 30 Days

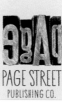

PAGE STREET
PUBLISHING CO.

First published in 2016 by
Page Street Publishing Co.
27 Congress Street, Suite 103
Salem, MA 01970
www.pagestreetpublishing.com

Distributed by Macmillan, sales in Canada by The Canadian Manda Group.

19 18 17 16   1 2 3 4 5

ISBN-13: 9781624142123
ISBN-10: 1624142125

Library of Congress Control Number: 2015943257

Cover and book design by Page Street Publishing Co.
Cover Image: Getty Images

Printed and bound in China

Page Street is proud to be a member of 1% for the Planet. Members donate one percent of their sales to one or more of the over 1,500 environmental and sustainability charities across the globe who participate in this program.

This book is dedicated to Gram.

CONTENTS

FOREWORD
by Michael Bergman, MD

There is a worldwide crisis of obesity and diabetes today. The International Diabetes Federation (IDF) estimates that 8.3 percent of the world's population, or 387 million individuals, have diabetes and 592 million, or 1 in 10, are expected to develop diabetes by 2035.[1] By the year 2050, it is estimated that 1 in 3 will have diabetes in conjunction with an aging population.[2] In addition, 316 million are considered at high risk for developing diabetes (prediabetes), with an expectation that this will increase to 500 million within a generation.[3]

Prediabetes defines a blood sugar level that is higher than normal but not sufficiently elevated to be classified as type 2 diabetes. There are currently 86 million individuals with prediabetes, affecting 1 in 3 Americans. Without intervention, prediabetes may evolve to type 2 diabetes within ten years. Furthermore, the long-term complications typically associated with diabetes, such as eye disease, may already be present with prediabetes. It is highly encouraging to note, however, that this situation may be reversible if prediabetes or diabetes is diagnosed sufficiently early and by incorporating changes in lifestyle to include healthier eating, increasing physical activity and maintaining a desirable weight.

Furthermore, medication is often not required when prediabetes is detected at a very early stage; a variety of clinical studies have consistently documented that lifestyle changes involving a weight-loss goal of 7 percent with a minimum of 150 minutes per week of exercise can be almost twice as effective as the use of drugs for the treatment of prediabetes. For those with diabetes who are already receiving medication, adopting a healthier lifestyle can lead to a reduction or elimination in the use of medication. Although prevention is the primary objective, it is never too late to improve glucose control by changes in therapeutic lifestyle.

Forty percent of adults face a lifetime risk of diabetes, representing a substantial increase from 20 percent in the late 1980s.[4] Delaying the diagnosis can result in at least one complication by the time an individual has been diagnosed. These statistics are particularly disturbing as more than 70 percent of cases, approximating 150 million cases by the year 2035,[5] can be delayed or prevented by adopting a healthier lifestyle. Furthermore, up to 11 percent of total health-care expenditures in every country could be reduced by addressing risk factors for type 2 diabetes.[6]

The 28-Day Blood Sugar Miracle, authored by Cher Pastore, MS, RD, CDE, a prominent, highly experienced dietitian/nutritionist and certified diabetes educator, is a clear, focused, easy-to-follow and practical guide to enhanced nutrition with a primary emphasis on plant-derived foods. Considerable research and effort has gone into providing an easy-to-comprehend book, including a clear, lucid, inviting and palatable scientific background, making this most appealing. Many diet books are extreme, faddist and therefore short-lived. What has been lacking, which separates this book from others, is a simple, intuitive, mainstream and logical approach to better eating and living, which can result in sustained weight loss and blood sugar control.

Cher's guidelines to better health are well-balanced, realistic, pragmatic and easy to incorporate. This book abounds with real-life examples of developing more nutritious and healthier eating habits, whether at home or out. Her recommendations are not theoretical or vague, but contain specific and detailed diet plans with abundant, tasteful menu options based on scientific study and many years of experience in helping her patients lose weight and control/prevent or reverse their diabetes. Considerable effort has gone into developing regimens that are not only healthy, but exciting, appealing and offering variety. This book will not only be of value to those with metabolic disorders, but will genuinely benefit everyone who is health conscious and seeking a more nutritious lifestyle.

—**Michael Bergman, MD, FACP,** NYU School of Medicine, Clinical Professor of Medicine, Director, NYU Diabetes Prevention Program

INTRODUCTION

I want to cry every time a patient sits in front of me and tells me they have just been diagnosed with type 2 diabetes. But I don't. I sit quietly and keep my calm as I listen to their story. I have to be strong. I am there to help them—I just wish they had come to me sooner.

According to the American Diabetes Association (ADA), over 29 million people, 9.3 percent of the population, have diabetes in the United States.[7] An additional 86 million US residents suffer from prediabetes. That's a third of the US population grappling with a disease designated as the leading cause of kidney failure, blindness and amputation, a key driver of heart disease and the seventh-leading cause of death in the United States. According to the Centers for Disease Control and Prevention (CDC), 1 in 3 people will have diabetes by 2050.[8]

I'm Cher Pastore, a registered dietitian (RD) and a certified diabetes educator (CDE) with a master's degree in nutrition and over 15 years of focused education and training in nutrition and the science of diabetes. As a seasoned entrepreneur with a successful private practice, I have helped many clients take control of their diabetes, lose weight and transition to living a healthier life. I also counsel clients on a variety of other health issues, including, but not limited to, prenatal and maternal nutrition, cardiovascular disease, digestive problems and thyroid disorders.

This is what I do—I help people improve their life through healthy eating. I meet with patients on a daily basis to help them prevent, reverse or control their diabetes through dietary and lifestyle modifications. Scientists confirm that by adopting a plant-based diet and making lifestyle changes, many diseases of the 21st century can be prevented.

Many of the problems that face Americans today stem from the food supply and the abundance of overly processed, chemically laden foods that line the shelves of the supermarket. It upsets me so much that consumers cannot go to a supermarket without being bombarded by false claims that a product is healthy, when in fact it is filled with ingredients that are not even recognizable, and sugar is a main component. Something must be done about this problem.

This is why I wrote *The 28-Day Blood Sugar Miracle*. The Blood Sugar Miracle (BSM) way of life is the result of my passion for healthy eating, my experience counseling patients on nutrition and diabetes management, and the success I have seen my patients achieve during my ten years as a private practitioner. One day I put them all together and the Blood Sugar Miracle—a whole foods, plant-based way of life for preventing, treating and beating diabetes—was born.

Through the years I have tried different approaches to helping my clients control their blood sugar—from carbohydrate counting, to portion control, to a low-carbohydrate/high-protein diet—all with some elements of success. However, once I started doing research on a plant-based diet as a way to treat diabetes, I became intrigued. I began trying it out with many of my clients. The results were staggering. The clients I put on a plant-based diet saw a significant drop in their blood sugar in the least amount of time as opposed to those on other diets! When my clients transitioned from eating a highly processed diet, including meat, to the Blood Sugar Miracle way of eating, they reported that they didn't feel hungry, lowered their glucose levels, had more energy, were able to think more clearly and lost weight more easily.

Unhealthy Eating and Me . . . and How Everything Changed

Before I go further into things, let me tell you about my journey with food and what led me to become a dietitian and a diabetes educator.

I grew up just like every other kid—eating junk food. Pizza, chips, cookies, cheeseburgers, TV dinners and soda, just to name a few, were staples in my diet. I vividly remember many days in high school when, unbeknownst to my parents, my lunch consisted of chocolate chip cookies and potato chips (cringe)! I ate like this for years. In fact, my house was the "junk food" house. All of my friends would say, "Let's go to your house after school; you have the best snacks." Meaning, chips and cookies and more! I never realized what it was doing to me and what the implications of eating like that had on my health. I wondered why I often didn't feel well, frequently got sick and didn't have enough energy—although I never connected it to what I was eating.

I was in my last year of high school when my life took a different path. Ever since I was a young girl, I knew I wanted to help people. I wanted to do something involving science, but I didn't know exactly what that was— until my grandfather, with whom I was very close, was diagnosed with lung cancer.

By the time we found out his diagnosis, his cancer was very advanced. However, he decided to undergo a course of treatment that included chemotherapy. During the course of treatments, he lost interest in eating. Over the next year, I went to all his treatment sessions with him and witnessed firsthand the effect that a lack of food has on a person's overall well-being. He had no energy, he was lackluster, his mood was down and he was losing a ton of weight. He was basically wasting away. He couldn't eat, but I knew that he needed food to give him strength for chemotherapy—and to beat cancer! I started reading about what foods were easier for him to tolerate and making all his meals, which in turn helped him eat.

That year my life changed. Before this, I didn't think much about what I ate myself and in fact, my diet was pretty poor—full of processed and sugar-laden junk foods, as I mentioned earlier. During that year of making meals for my grandfather, I made the connection that the food we put in our bodies is where it all starts. I decided then that I wanted to help people who were struggling with diseases such as cancer or diabetes. So, I went on a mission to learn all that I could about the science of nutrition and how the right foods give us energy, contribute to a healthy lifestyle and help fight disease(s).

I learned quickly that proper nutrition is vital before, during and after cancer treatments: that what you eat directly affects how you feel, what diseases you can potentially avoid or reverse; and how the right foods help control your weight. In short, I realized the healing power of food.

What had started out as something so negative turned into a positive experience. I realized what I wanted to do with the rest of my life, and I have been helping people eat better and improve their lives through proper nutrition every day since then.

First, I used what I had learned on myself. It was that year that I also stopped eating red meat (my parents were horrified). I instantly started to feel better. I also stopped drinking soda and cut down on (although didn't stop eating) junk food. That was a more gradual transition, however. When I went to college and began studying nutrition further, I changed the way I ate even more. I became an official vegetarian in college and started making my own meals. I was very happy with the way I felt and how I was eating. It wasn't until years later that I took it even further and embraced plant-based eating. To this day, the way I eat continues to evolve, with the constant goal of living the healthiest life that I can.

Why the Blood Sugar Miracle Was Born

The American Academy of Nutrition and Dietetics and the American Diabetes Association both recommend well-planned, plant-based (vegetarian or vegan) nutrition for people with diabetes.[9] Even the US Department of Agriculture (USDA)'s 2010 Dietary Guidelines for Americans showed praise for a plant-based diet.[10] Dietary Guidelines are released every five years. The 2015 Dietary Guidelines Advisory Committee submitted the Scientific Report of the 2015 Dietary Guidelines Advisory Committee to the secretaries of the US Department of Health and Human Services (HHS) and the USDA in February 2015. It reported that "major findings regarding sustainable diets were that a diet higher in plant-based foods, such as vegetables, fruits, whole grains, legumes, nuts and seeds, and lower in calories and animal-based foods is more health promoting and is associated with less environmental impact than is the current US diet."[11] As this book went to press, the official 2015 Dietary Guidelines were not yet released.

Clinical research studies have shown that adopting a low-fat, plant-derived diet can help reverse a type 2 diabetes diagnosis. Whole plant foods can improve insulin sensitivity, aid in weight loss, contribute to a healthy intestinal track and reduce blood sugar and cholesterol. Additionally, heart disease, the #1 killer in the United States, was found to be almost nonexistent in populations with a foundation in plant-based diets. A plant-based diet may also help in preventing or slowing certain cancers. This is mostly because whole plant foods contain antioxidants that fight against aging and cancer. Basically, plant-based nutrition leads to a longer life.

In addition, certain foods, specifically those containing magnesium, biotin, chromium and omega-3s, are good for diabetics. What are good and bad carbohydrates? How does a plant-based diet provide more energy? These solutions are addressed and then applied in food recommendations and recipes throughout the book. The recipes are nutrient balanced, to include plenty of plant-based protein sources. With the understanding that some people can't practice a strict vegan diet, some fish and egg options are included in Phase 2 of the plan. Even desserts can't be completely avoided, so I have included some scrumptious, easy-to-prepare desserts for those with a sweet tooth.

The Blood Sugar Miracle is more than just a diet. It is a whole foods, plant-based way of life that transforms people from the inside out. The BSM provides an organized nutrition plan for people who have diabetes, as well as for those who are prediabetic and those who want to prevent diabetes or reverse their type 2 diabetes diagnosis. A plant-based approach has also proven successful for those who are suffering from chronic disease, such as hypertension, heart disease and obesity. The Blood Sugar Miracle is also ideal for vegetarians who want to take it to the next level and become vegan, those who want to lose weight in general and anyone who wants to eat healthier and help the environment at the same time.

Stop destroying your health. Stop obesity and diabetes.

When you stop eating overly processed foods and large quantities of added sugar, you will be thinner, healthier and happier.

Come along with me on this journey. I have done it, my patients have done it and you can do it, too.

Lower Your Blood Sugar, Lose Weight, Reverse Diabetes and Change Your Life in 28 Days

In *The 28-Day Blood Sugar Miracle*, I will show you how to:

1. Decrease your sugar cravings

2. Learn to eat whole, natural, nutritious foods

3. Understand once and for all the truth about carbohydrates

4. Follow a way of life that will leave you satisfied and transform your body

5. Prepare easy, delicious and healthy recipes

Trust me, in 28 days you will be off processed foods, thinner and feeling better. Once you adopt this way of life and keep up with its healthy habits, you can prevent obesity and diabetes or potentially reverse a type 2 diabetes diagnosis.

Let's get started!

CHAPTER 1

THE BLOOD SUGAR MIRACLE—A DIET WITH A PURPOSE

1. Do you have diabetes or prediabetes?

2. Do you want to lower your blood sugar?

3. Do you have intense cravings for sugar?

4. Do you have excess weight that you want to lose?

5. Do you want to feel better and more energetic?

If you answered *yes* to any of these questions, now is the time to take action.

THE PROBLEM WITH THE TYPICAL AMERICAN DIET

The first problem with the typical American diet is too many calories. In the days of "too busy to cook" and "not enough time" for balanced meals, Americans rely too much on fast food, frozen meals and liquid nourishment because they are more convenient. If only we transferred the time spent in front of the TV or online, we could easily find more time for nutritious meals.

The typical meal in America today is filled with an overabundance of refined grains, foods with added sugar and fats, meat and poultry. Although the typical American family in the 1950s sat down to dinners of meat, potatoes and vegetables, it was simple. Meals were primarily eaten at home, or came from home or a restaurant. Everywhere we go today, food is readily available and is associated with almost every social activity. You can buy snacks or meals at roadside rest stops, sports games, convenience stores, even gyms and health clubs. Book clubs, business meetings and even youth sleepovers are coupled with something to munch on. When we are bored, stressed out or want to celebrate, food is involved.

Americans are also spending far more on foods eaten outside of the home. In 1970, we spent 27 percent of our food budget on away-from-home food; by 2006, that percentage had risen to 46 percent. Americans are also obsessed with "supersizing" it, thinking they are getting more for their money. They are also adding more to their waistline, but most don't realize it until it creates a health problem.

Data from the National Health and Nutrition Examination Survey (NHANES), 2011–2012, indicates that more than a third of US adults over age 20 are overweight or obese, and 6.4 percent are extremely obese.[12] Results also showed that 16.9 percent of US children and adolescents ages 2–19 years are obese and 14.9 percent are overweight.[13] Physical inactivity and obesity are common catalysts for the development of insulin resistance, prediabetes and type 2 diabetes.

What Is Insulin Resistance and What Causes It?

Insulin is a hormone that is made by the pancreas and gets secreted in response to glucose entering the bloodstream. Insulin aids in blood sugar control in three ways: (1) It helps muscle, fat and liver cells absorb glucose from the bloodstream, (2) it helps the liver and muscle store excess sugar (glycogen) and (3) it reduces glucose production in the liver.[14]

Insulin resistance is a condition in which your body produces insulin but does not use it effectively. Thus, if you have insulin resistance, it causes sugar to build up in the bloodstream. The major causes of insulin resistance appear to be excess weight (especially around the waist) and physical inactivity.

How Insulin Resistance Leads to Prediabetes and Type 2 Diabetes

If you have not already been diagnosed with diabetes, you may not even know that you have insulin resistance. Most people won't even know they have insulin resistance until it turns into full-blown type 2 diabetes. Normally, there are no symptoms of insulin resistance. So, you can have insulin resistance or prediabetes for several years without knowing it. This, in turn, can lead to type 2 diabetes, unless you make some lifestyle changes. The only way to confirm whether you have insulin resistance, prediabetes or type 2 diabetes is to get tested by your doctor. Insulin resistance can be only be assessed by measuring the level of insulin in the blood. In addition to diabetes, insulin resistance can lead to other serious health disorders, including cardiovascular disease, nonalcoholic fatty liver disease and chronic kidney disease.

What Is Diabetes and How Many Types Are There?

Diabetes is a group of diseases marked by high levels of blood glucose resulting from defects in insulin production, insulin action or both. There are four primary forms of diabetes.

Type 1: Type 1 diabetes develops when the body's immune system destroys pancreatic beta cells, which are the only cells in the body that make the hormone insulin that regulates blood glucose. To survive, people with type 1 diabetes must have insulin delivered by an exogenous source, such as injection, pump or inhaler.

Type 2: Type 2 diabetes accounts for 90 to 95 percent of all diagnosed diabetes cases.[15] Type 2 diabetes usually begins as insulin resistance. As the need for insulin rises, the pancreas gradually loses its ability to produce insulin. Type 2 diabetes (non-insulin-dependent diabetes mellitus, or NIDDM), previously referred to as adult-onset diabetes, is being diagnosed more frequently among children and adolescents, with obesity as the main catalyst.

Gestational diabetes: Gestational diabetes is a form of glucose intolerance diagnosed during pregnancy. Five to 10 percent of women continue to have high blood glucose levels after pregnancy and are diagnosed as having diabetes, usually type 2. Children of women who had gestational diabetes during pregnancies may also be at risk of developing obesity and diabetes.

Prediabetes: Currently, 79 million US residents suffer from prediabetes. Those with prediabetes have glucose levels higher than normal, but not high enough to be classified as diabetes. According to the CDC,[16] without lifestyle changes, 15 to 30 percent of people with prediabetes will develop type 2 diabetes within five years.

How Important Is Blood Sugar and What Should Your Blood Sugar Be?

Blood sugar, also known as blood glucose, is the concentration of glucose in the blood—the sugar transported through blood that provides energy to the cells in the body. The human body converts carbohydrates into glucose, which is a simple sugar that your body can easily convert to energy. Glucose is the primary source of energy in the human body.

After food intake, blood sugar concentration rises and the pancreas releases insulin to ensure that glucose enters the cells to give us energy. Without insulin in the bloodstream, no glucose gets into the cells, and they can starve. You know how you feel when you haven't eaten in a while. No energy, right? This is otherwise known as low blood sugar, or hypoglycemia. When blood glucose levels drop, the pancreas releases glucagon, which triggers the breakdown of glycogen into glucose and increases the blood glucose levels back to normal. Excess glucose (as glycogen) is stored in the muscles and the liver.

In the body of a nondiabetic person, glucose levels are automatically regulated to maintain the stability necessary for the body to function. In a diabetic person, blood sugar levels are too high, also known as hyperglycemia, which can be caused by several things—the pancreas does not make enough insulin, cells do not respond to insulin normally or both. In type 1 diabetics, the body either produces too little or no insulin, and insulin injections are required. In type 2 diabetics, the same situation is true, but blood sugar can be controlled with the right food intake.

Type 2 diabetics account for a majority of diabetes diagnoses. The best, long-range solution for controlling blood sugar is a well-planned, balanced and monitored diet, which is essential for insulin management. The Blood Sugar Miracle will help prevent those highs and lows.

The average blood glucose level in the human body is about 90 mg/dL (milligrams per deciliter), which is equivalent to 5 mM (millimoles per liter). Normal ranges are from 90 to 120 mg/dL.

All diabetics are susceptible to both hyperglycemia and hypoglycemia, so monitoring of blood glucose levels on a regular basis is important.

When Should You Check Your Blood Sugar?

How often you check your blood sugar depends on the type of diabetes you have and whether you are insulin dependent. However, the main times to check your blood sugar are before and after you eat, before and after you are physically active and before you go to sleep.

FOR GESTATIONAL DIABETICS, YOUR GLUCOSE LEVEL SHOULD BE:

1. 90 mg/dL or less, upon waking (after fasting 8 hours)
2. 140 mg/dL or less one hour after a meal
3. 120 mg/dL or less two hours after a meal

FOR TYPE 2 DIABETICS, YOUR GLUCOSE LEVEL SHOULD BE:

1. 70–100 mg/dL, upon waking (after fasting 8 hours)
2. 100–140 mg/dL, two hours after a meal

Note—Your exact regimen should be discussed with your medical doctor, endocrinologist or certified diabetes educator.

Are You at Risk for Prediabetes and Type 2 Diabetes?

While researchers don't fully understand why some people develop type 2 diabetes and others don't, it is clear that certain factors increase your risk for developing the disease, including:

Obesity—Being overweight presents a high risk factor for type 2 diabetes. The more fat tissue you have, the harder it is for your body to use insulin. Additionally, if you have more body fat around your midsection, your risk is greater than if your extra fat is stored elsewhere.

Your lifestyle—Poor diet and lack of physical activity can lead to obesity. Regular physical activity helps control your weight and helps your body process glucose normally and use insulin better. The less exercise you get, the greater your risk.

Your family history—While most cases of type 1 diabetes are attributed to hereditary factors from parents, type 2 diabetes has a stronger connection to family history than does type 1. That connection strongly depends on environmental factors, such as lifestyle (which involves nutrition and exercise). Poor eating and exercise habits tend to run in families that have a common upbringing. These habits can contribute to obesity.

Race—People of certain races—including African Americans, Hispanics, American Indians and Asian Americans—are more likely to develop type 2 diabetes than are Caucasian Americans.

Age—The risk of type 2 diabetes increases after age 45.

Prediabetes—If you have prediabetes, then you are at a very high risk for developing type 2 diabetes.

Gestational diabetes—If you developed gestational diabetes during pregnancy, you are at an increased risk of getting type 2 diabetes later in your life.

How to Tell if You Have Prediabetes or Type 2 Diabetes

If you think you may be at risk for prediabetes or type 2 diabetes, take the appropriate risk test below. If you score less than 9 on the prediabetes test or more than 5 on the type 2 diabetes risk test, consult your primary care physician. Only your doctor can officially diagnose diabetes, prescribe additional testing if needed and refer you to a certified diabetes educator for diabetes-specific nutrition education.

The easiest way to diagnose diabetes is with the A1c test, which is a simple blood test performed at your doctor's office. The A1c test reflects your average blood sugar level for the past two to three months. If your A1c has a value of 6.5 percent or higher, then you have diabetes.

BLOOD TEST LEVELS FOR DIABETES DIAGNOSIS	
Diagnosis	**A1c Level**
Diabetes	6.5 percent or above
Prediabetes	5.7 to 6.4 percent
Normal	4 to 5.6 percent

But, if you are diagnosed with type 2 diabetes, all is not lost! The Blood Sugar Miracle plan can help you reverse the type 2 diagnosis. While hereditary factors are not controllable, the BSM plan will help you to take control, so you can combat the risk factors and live a healthier life.

CDC PREDIABETES SCREENING TEST*
COULD YOU HAVE PREDIABETES?

Prediabetes means your blood glucose (sugar) is higher than normal, but not yet diabetes. Diabetes is a serious disease that can cause heart attack, stroke, blindness, kidney failure, or loss of feet or legs. Type 2 diabetes can be delayed or prevented in people with prediabetes through effective lifestyle programs. Take the first step. Find out your risk for prediabetes.

TAKE THE TEST—KNOW YOUR SCORE!

Answer these seven simple questions. For each "Yes" answer, add the number of points listed. All "No" answers are 0 points.

- Are you a woman who has had a baby weighing more than 9 pounds at birth? (1)
- Do you have a sister or brother with diabetes? (1)
- Do you have a parent with diabetes? (1)
- Find your height on the chart (next page). Do you weigh as much as or more than the weight listed for your height? (5)
- Are you younger than 65 years of age and get little or no exercise in a typical day? (5)
- Are you between 45 and 64 years of age? (5)
- Are you 65 years of age or older? (9)

Add your score and check the next page to see what it means.

*Courtesy of the American Diabetes Association

AT-RISK WEIGHT CHART	
Height	**Weight (Pounds)**
4'10"	129
4'11"	133
5'0"	138
5'1"	143
5'2"	147
5'3"	152
5'4"	157
5'5"	162
5'6"	167
5'7"	172
5'8"	177
5'9"	182
5'10"	188
5'11"	193
6'0"	199
6'1"	204
6'2"	210
6'3"	216
6'4"	221

IF YOUR SCORE IS 3 TO 8 POINTS

This means your risk is probably low for having prediabetes now. Keep your risk low. If you're overweight, lose weight. Be active most days, and don't use tobacco. Eat low-fat meals with fruits, vegetables and whole-grain foods. If you have high cholesterol or high blood pressure, talk to your health-care provider about your risk for type 2 diabetes.

IF YOUR SCORE IS 9 OR MORE POINTS

This means your risk is high for having prediabetes now. Please make an appointment with your health-care provider soon.

HOW CAN I GET TESTED FOR PREDIABETES?

Individual or group health insurance: See your health-care provider. If you don't have a provider, ask your insurance company about providers who take your insurance. Deductibles and copays may apply.

Medicaid: See your health-care provider. If you don't have a provider, contact a state Medicaid office or contact your local health department.

Medicare: See your health-care provider. Medicare will pay the cost of testing if the provider has a reason for testing. If you don't have a provider, contact your local health department.

No insurance: Contact your local health department for more information about where you could be tested or call your local health clinic.

ARE YOU AT RISK FOR TYPE 2 DIABETES?

Diabetes Risk Test*

1. How old are you?

   ❑ Less than 40 years (0 points)

   ❑ 40—49 years (1 point)

   ❑ 50—59 years (2 points)

   ❑ 60 years or older (3 points)

2. Are you a man or a woman?

   ❑ Man (1 point)

   ❑ Woman (0 points)

3. If you are a woman, have you ever been diagnosed with gestational diabetes?

   ❑ Yes (1 point)

   ❑ No (0 points)

4. Do you have a mother, father, sister or brother with diabetes?

   ❑ Yes (1 point)

   ❑ No (0 points)

5. Have you ever been diagnosed with high blood pressure?

   ❑ Yes (1 point)

   ❑ No (0 points)

6. Are you physically active?

   ❑ Yes (0 points)

   ❑ No (1 point)

*Courtesy of the Centers for Disease and Prevention Control, Diabetes Prevention Program

(continued)

7. What is your weight status? (see chart)

HEIGHT	WEIGHT (POUNDS)		
4'10"	119–142	143–190	191+
4'11"	124–147	148–197	198+
5'0"	128–152	153–203	204+
5'1"	132–157	158–210	211+
5'2"	136–163	164–217	218+
5'3"	141–168	169–224	225+
5'4"	145–173	174–231	232+
5'5"	150–179	180–239	240+
5'6"	155–185	186–246	247+
5'7"	159–190	191–254	255+
5'8"	164–196	197–261	262+
5'9"	169–202	203–269	270+
5'10"	174–208	209–277	278+
5'11"	179–214	215–285	286+
6'0"	184–220	221–293	294+
6'1"	189–226	227–301	302+
6'2"	194–232	233–310	311+
6'3"	200–239	240–318	319+
6'4"	205–245	246–327	328+
	(1 Point)	(2 Points)	(3 Points)
You weigh less than the amount in the left column (0 points)			

If you scored 5 or higher: You are at increased risk for having type 2 diabetes. However, only your doctor can tell for sure if you do have type 2 diabetes or prediabetes (a condition that precedes type 2 diabetes in which blood glucose levels are higher than normal). Talk to your doctor to see if additional testing is needed.

Type 2 diabetes is more common in African Americans, Hispanics/Latinos, American Indians, Asian Americans and Pacific Islanders. Higher body weights increase diabetes risk for everyone. Asian Americans are at increased diabetes risk at lower body weights than the rest of the general public (about 15 pounds lower).

For more information, visit us at diabetes.org/alert or call 1-800-DIABETES (1-800-342-2383).

Lower Your Risk

The good news is that you can manage your risk for type 2 diabetes. Small steps make a big difference and can help you live a longer, healthier life.

If you are at high risk, your first step is to see your doctor to see if additional testing is needed.

Visit diabetes.org or call 1-800-DIABETES (1-800-342-2383) for information, tips on getting started and ideas for simple, small steps you can take to help lower your risk.

WHAT IS THE BLOOD SUGAR MIRACLE?

The Blood Sugar Miracle way of life was born through my passion for healthy eating, my experience counseling clients on nutrition and diabetes management, and the success I have seen my clients achieve during my 10 years as a private practitioner. I have helped many clients take control of their diabetes, lose weight and transition to living a healthier life.

On a daily basis clients ask me, "Can I eat carbs?" "Can I eat fruit?" "What fruit should I eat?" "What about desserts?" "Do I need to count calories?" "How can I get enough protein without eating meat?" "What about exercise?" "Can I have a glass of wine or a beer?" It occurred to me that people are not clear on what to eat in order to control their blood sugar, whether they can safely "cheat" and how to lose weight without fad diets, gimmicks or surgery. With busy schedules and the presence of quick, cheap, easy meals on the go, obesity is no surprise. Processed foods are cheaper, but contain toxic ingredients. Going "vegan" sounds too extreme to some people. Education is a key component for diabetes care and prevention. Understanding calorie and portion control, staple foods that aid in glucose stability, the importance of eating whole foods and plant-based nutrition are all part of the Blood Sugar Miracle.

For anyone who needs—and wants—direction and guidance on basic nutrition, an easy-to-understand daily nutrition plan and easy recipes to help fulfill that plan, the Blood Sugar Miracle is the answer.

Why You Need to Eat This Way to Control Your Blood Sugar

Processed or refined foods, such as white bread, fast foods and liquid meals often contain more sugar and break down faster. These types of foods cause a spike in blood sugar, which also results in a crash shortly thereafter. Plant-based diets include foods that have high fiber content, which help control cravings by providing a steady stream of nutrition—so your body avoids the sugar highs and lows. Plant-based diets also help lower blood cholesterol levels, the risk of heart disease, blood pressure levels and the risk of hypertension and type 2 diabetes.

The Added Benefit of Weight Loss

People who follow a plant-based diet tend to have a lower body mass index (BMI), representing a higher lean muscle to fat ratio, which translates to a better body composition and a higher metabolism overall.

When you eat whole foods, your body has to expend energy to break down that food and process it. Did you ever wonder why you feel heated after eating? That is your metabolism on fire, breaking down what you just ate. Fad diets that include fasting and liquid meals have an adverse effect on the human body. When you "drink" a meal, your body doesn't have to do anything to process it. So, your metabolism just cruises along, not getting revved up at all.

The same goes for eating regular meals throughout the day, versus one big meal a day. The human body can only digest so many calories per meal and the overage goes to your fat cells for storage. Every time you eat, your metabolism is kicked into gear. Eating on a regular basis keeps your metabolism revved throughout the day. The Blood Sugar Miracle plan provides the right balance of carbs, protein and fat to keep your energy up throughout the day.

A Diet That Will Become a Way of Life

When people begin a plant-based diet, most see dramatic improvements in weight, cholesterol and blood sugar. The need for medications diminishes, and some may not need medications at all. "But what about the cost?" you ask. The money you invest in eating whole foods now will reduce the future health care costs on medication and doctor visits related to poor health. The Blood Sugar Miracle aims to improve your health from the inside out! It also gives you an easy-to-follow plan, complete with recipes and nutrition information and provides guidance to help you choose wisely when eating outside the home.

BRIAN'S STORY
I now have control of my blood sugar, and I lost 30 pounds in the process!

I have been overweight my whole life. I used to emotionally eat. I grew up as the fat kid in New York City and after years of not exercising and eating too much, I developed diabetes. I knew it was coming—my doctor warned me. She told me that if I didn't start eating right and losing some weight, I was going to develop type 2 diabetes. But I didn't listen. I kept eating the way I normally did. Bagels for breakfast, sandwiches for lunch and every night I would order take-out and have it delivered. Both the Chinese and pizza delivery guys knew my name and order. Looking back now, it was pretty pathetic. I was depressed and I couldn't see my way out. How was I going to make these changes? It seemed overwhelming. The pounds kept piling on and on, and my blood sugar became out of control. I had no energy, I was tired and hungry all the time and I was miserable. At that point I was up to 290 pounds. It seemed so much easier to just keep doing what I was doing. Until it was too late.

I started getting all of the symptoms; I was thirsty and urinating all of the time. I knew something was wrong. I made an appointment with my doctor, and she said I had diabetes. She immediately referred me to Cher, and she and I started working together. But my blood sugar numbers were pretty high, so I had to start taking oral medication. Cher put me on the Blood Sugar Miracle diet. When she told me for the first 28 days I had to cut out all animal products, I thought there is no way I can do this: I love to eat steak and hamburgers, and I definitely won't be able to stop eating cheese.

But I did it. It wasn't as hard as I thought it was going to be. At first I thought, How am I going to do this? How am I going to live without hamburgers, bagels with cream cheese, Chinese food, pizza?! I really didn't know. But I started—just as Cher told me to do.

I just followed the plan, and it was a miracle—I instantly started to feel better. All of the cravings that I was having disappeared, and I wasn't hungry. I started to have more energy, and I really liked this new way of eating.

I was still able to order Chinese food. I just ordered it differently—now I order mixed vegetables with tofu with a small amount of brown rice, instead of egg rolls and pork lo mein. I am still able to go out to dinner with my family and friends—I just order differently. It doesn't feel like a hardship because I am feeling so much better.

I started eating like this well over a year ago, and I have lost 30 pounds, I have lowered my blood sugar and I have gotten off all of my medications. Before I was dying—now I am living.

How Can the Blood Sugar Miracle Help You?

If you are diabetic, at risk for being diagnosed with diabetes, diabetes is hereditary in your family, or you have chronic health problems such as obesity, hypertension or cardiovascular disease, The Blood Sugar Miracle can help you. Most people diagnosed with diabetes did not know they had it until a symptom of the disease appeared. Don't let it get that far. Be proactive and start eating the right way now.

Following the Blood Sugar Miracle will help you to reverse a type 2 diagnosis and other chronic health issues, such as high cholesterol, cardiovascular disease, hypertension and obesity. Low-fat, plant-based eating patterns have been effective in reducing LDL cholesterol concentrations, which result in significant reductions in cardiovascular disease risk and cardiovascular events. Studies of hypertension found that those abstaining from all animal products achieved the most significant improvements in lowering blood pressure and hypertension.[15] Comparative studies of adults practicing nonvegan versus vegan diets have also shown a lower prevalence of type 2 diabetes, cardiovascular disease and obesity, and reduced medical care usage with those on vegan diets.

The Blood Sugar Miracle is high in fiber and water, resulting in higher satiety and reduced cravings for added calories above the recommended daily intake. You will have more energy and lose fat, which will result in overall weight loss and better health!

To-Do List

1. Take the assesment tests—A CDC Prediabetes Screening Test (page 17) or Are You At Risk for Type 2 Diabetes? (page 19).

2. Go meatless one day per week.

3. Cut out all artificial sweeteners.

4. Start cutting out all added sugar.

CHAPTER 2

THE TRUTH ABOUT CARBOHYDRATES

My patients are always asking me about carbohydrates—or "carbs." Can I eat carbs? Can I eat fruit? Doesn't fruit have a lot of sugar? Which carbs can I have? Low- or no-carb diets, such as Atkins, Dukan and even the currently popular Paleo diet are targeted for quick weight loss and are not healthy in the long term.

On low-carb diets, if your body uses up its carb stores, it can turn to fat stores for energy. But that is not a long-term solution. While fats can be a source of energy for most of the body, a few types of cells, such as brain cells, can't run on fatty acids directly. I'm sure you've experienced being ineffective or unproductive when you are hungry. Your brain needs carbs, too!

Carbs are not the enemy! Consuming too many carbs is, however. Especially if you are consuming too many processed foods, which are full of calories, bad carbs (sugar) and high levels of fat. Some carbs are healthier than others, and you have to know how much your body requires. Proper blood sugar control depends on knowing which carbs to select and how much! Here is the truth about carbs—once and for all.

WHAT IS A CARBOHYDRATE?

A carbohydrate is one of the necessary macronutrients, along with protein and fat, which our bodies require for energy. When you think about carbs, think energy—carbs are the body's primary source of fuel (followed by protein and fat, in that order). Carbs are found mainly in fruits, vegetables, dairy and grains—foods that are made up of sugar, starches and fiber.

Carbs have the largest impact on your blood sugar. Carbs break down into sugar in the body, which in turn provides you with energy. When you think about how many carbohydrates to eat on a daily basis, think about how much physical activity and exercise you will be getting that day. If you are going to be driving in your car and then sitting at your desk all day, then you aren't really going to need to consume a high amount of carbs that day. If you are going to be physically active and getting at least 60 minutes of exercise that day, then your body requires a bit more. Consuming more carbs than your body needs on a daily basis leads to obesity, which can lead to insulin resistance, which can lead to diabetes.

How Carbohydrates Are Metabolized in the Body

When you eat carbs, they are metabolized in your body both as a carbohydrate (sugar) and as a fat. After you ingest carbs, the sugar transforms into fructose and glucose. Glucose, or blood sugar, is stored as glycogen in your muscles and liver, and your body draws on this for short-term energy. The remaining glucose (about 80 percent) goes into the bloodstream for use by the cells in your body. If there is leftover glucose beyond what the liver can hold, it can be turned into fat storage for use later. Fructose, a sugar found naturally in many fruits and vegetables, and added to various beverages, such as soda and fruit-flavored drinks, is metabolized through your liver and mostly converted to fat and stored for later use.

Every cell in your body requires glucose to survive, which is why your blood sugar levels are so important. Carbs can only be stored in limited quantities, so your body needs them at regular intervals to use them for energy.

Good Carbs vs. Bad Carbs

The way carbs are broken down in the body is what makes a carb more or less desirable. Some carbs break down quickly—you want to avoid these—some take longer to break down and some don't digest at all, like certain fibers.

Carbohydrates are the largest group of food—they are found in nearly every food in your diet. They include such foods as bread, rice, pasta and cereals, as well as fruit, vegetables and dairy products. They also include processed foods, such as snacks, packaged foods and fast food, which tend to be filled with loads of sugar, fat and preservatives.

If a food has been highly processed—meaning many of its nutrients have been stripped— it will quickly turn into sugar in the body. When this happens, the glucose will enter your bloodstream rapidly, causing a spike in blood sugar. If you consume a large amount of these kinds of carbohydrates, it will lead to a large rise in blood sugar, which will then cause your body to produce insulin. If you continue to do this to your body over and over again, you will likely end up with insulin resistance, which is a precursor to diabetes.

More desirable carbohydrates include ones that take longer to digest. These include the starches that are found in whole-grain foods, beans and vegetables. Since starches take longer to metabolize than sugars, they have a time-release energy effect, and thus they will raise your blood sugar more slowly and offer more sustained energy levels.

The Worst Kind of Carb—Ultraprocessed Carbs (Avoid These!)

First, it is important to avoid anything that is highly processed. The biggest problem is ultraprocessed carbohydrates—they are in large part to blame for the obesity and diabetes crisis.

Recent studies show that processed foods are linked to many common diseases (diabetes, heart disease) as well as other health issues, including obesity.

The problem is not solely processed food but the extent to which the food is processed. According to new research, there are three levels of processed foods. Group 1 contains minimally processed foods. These include mostly whole foods that have been submitted to some form of processing without altering the nutritional properties of the food. Examples in this category are meats, grains, beans, milk and fresh fruits and vegetables. Group 2 contains substances extracted from whole foods. These include oil, fat, flour, pasta and sugar.[16] Group 3 is ultraprocessed foods, which include biscuits, cookies, breads, ice cream, cereal bars, chips, breakfast cereal and sugared soft drinks.

How can you tell if a food is minimally processed versus ultraprocessed? Let's look at an example.

Bread only needs to include flour, yeast (or an alternative), water and salt.

Here are the ingredients in Wonder Classic White Bread:

Wheat Flour Enriched (Flour, Barley Malt, Ferrous Sulfate [Iron], Vitamin B [Niacin], Vitamin B_3, Thiamine Mononitrate [Vitamin B_1], Riboflavin [Vitamin B_2], Folic Acid [Vitamin B_9]), Water, High-Fructose Corn Syrup, Contains 2% or less: Wheat Gluten, Salt, Soybean Oil, Yeast, Calcium Sulphate, Vinegar, Monoglyceride, Dough Conditioners (Sodium Stearoyl Lactylate, Calcium Dioxide), Soy Flour, Diammonium Phosphate, Dicalcium Phosphate, Monocalcium Phosphate, Yeast Nutrients (Ammonium Sulfate), Calcium Propionate, To Retain Freshness.

Now, I am not saying to eat homemade bread instead of Wonder Bread—or that you have to eat any bread at all. What I am saying is start looking at the ingredients in the foods that you are most commonly consuming, and start to omit the most amount of processed foods that you can.

The More Nutritious Carbohydrates (Choose These!)

Starches: Barley, beans and other legumes, a small sweet potato, quinoa, sprouted-grain toast

Vegetables: Alfalfa sprouts, arugula, asparagus, bamboo shoots, bell peppers (any color), broccoli, Brussels sprouts, cabbage, carrots, cauliflower, Chinese cabbage, chives, collard greens, cucumbers, daikon, eggplant, endive, escarole, garlic, green beans, jicama, kale, loose-leaf lettuce (red or green), mung bean sprouts, mushrooms, mustard greens, okra, onions, parsley, radicchio, radishes, romaine lettuce, spinach, Swiss chard, tomatoes, water chestnuts, watercress, yellow squash, zucchini

Fruits: 1 small apple, 1 cup (144 g) blackberries, 1 cup (148 g) blueberries, 2 kiwis, 1 nectarine, 1 small orange, 2 plums, 1 cup (123 g) raspberries, 6 large strawberries

HOW MANY CARBOHYDRATES DO YOU NEED?

For a typical inactive man eating 2,000 calories per day, I recommend 180 grams total of daily carbs. For a typical woman eating 1,800 calories per day, I recommend 150 grams total of carbohydrates. For a woman eating 1,200 calories per day, I recommend eating 120 grams of carbohydrates. For pregnant women, I recommend 150–175 grams of carbohydrates per day.

I recommend 30 to 50 grams per day of total dietary fiber.

Net carbohydrates are the grams of total carbohydrates in a portion of food minus its grams of fiber. Why are net carbohydrates important? Since fiber is not digested in the body, it does not raise your blood sugar levels or trigger an insulin response. However, if you are taking insulin, this calculation may be adjusted.

Also, if you are on a gluten-free diet, you can still follow the BSM plan. You will just avoid wheat, rye and barley, and you can use gluten-free oats. Here is a more detailed guideline for how much (good) carbohydrate you need on a daily basis:

FOOD GROUP	ALLOWED FOODS	SERVINGS PER DAY	SERVING SIZE	GRAMS OF CARBS PER SERVING	NUMBER OF SERVINGS PER DAY BASED ON DAILY CALORIC INTAKE OF:		
					1,200 CALORIES	1,600 CALORIES	2,000 CALORIES
Legumes	All beans: garbanzo (chickpeas), pinto, black, kidney, lima, navy, white; lentils; yellow and green split peas	1–3	½ cup cooked (about 100 g, depending on legume)	15	1	2	3
Vegetables	Arugula, artichokes, bamboo shoots, bell peppers, bok choy, broccoli, Brussels sprouts, cauliflower, celery, red cabbage, collard greens, cucumber, dandelion greens, eggplant, escarole, garlic, green beans, kale, leeks, lettuce, mixed greens, mushrooms, okra, onions, radishes, spinach, Swiss chard, tomatoes, watercress, zucchini	2–6	1 cup raw (about 230–340 g, depending on vegetable) or ½ cup cooked (about 90–135 g, depending on vegetable)	5	4	5	6

(continued)

FOOD GROUP	ALLOWED FOODS	SERVINGS PER DAY	SERVING SIZE	GRAMS OF CARBS PER SERVING	NUMBER OF SERVINGS PER DAY BASED ON DAILY CALORIC INTAKE OF:		
					1,200 CALORIES	1,600 CALORIES	2,000 CALORIES
Fruits	1 small apple, 1 cup blackberries (100 g), 1 cup blueberries (100 g), 2 clementines, 2 kiwis, 1 small orange, 2 plums, 1 cup raspberries (100 g), 6 large strawberries	2–3	Varies	15–20	2	2	3
Dairy (Phase 2)	1 ounce (28 g) regular cheese, low-fat cottage cheese, low-fat ricotta cheese, plain Greek yogurt	1	½ cup (115 g) to 1 cup (230 g)	7–15	1	1	1
Whole grains	Amaranth, barley, brown rice, buckwheat, millet, quinoa, spelt, sprouted-grain toast, whole oats, whole wheat, wild rice	1–3	1 slice bread, ½ cup (80 g) cooked grains, 3 rye crackers, 1 (6-inch [15-cm]) whole wheat tortilla	15	1	2	3

Carb Counting

How do you know how many carbohydrates you are eating? Well, if anything has a food label, you can just look right at it. On the label, look at the serving size and total grams of carbohydrates. And since you now know what a net carbohydrate is, you can also calculate the grams of net carbs.

If it doesn't have a label, then you can get a book on carb counting or look online. (See page 178 for resources on carbohydrate counting.)

Quiz: Are You Addicted to Carbs/Sugar?

1. Do you feel like you "have to have" something sweet after every meal?
2. Do you have strong cravings for sweets?
3. Do you use sweets as a reward?
4. Do you start to crave sweets if you are tired, bored or sad?
5. Does the thought of giving up sweets pose a challenge for you?
6. Have you ever taken a bite of something sweet and weren't able to stop eating it?
7. Have you given up sweets for a certain period of time and then binged on them?

If you answered yes to one or two of the questions, you are probably addicted to sugar. If you answered yes to more than two, then you are definitely addicted to sugar.

SUGAR SPIKER	WHY IT SPIKES SUGARS	GOOD SUBSTITUTES
White rice	All types of rice are very high in carbohydrates, the nutrient responsible for raising blood sugar. White rice in particular is bad because in addition to high carbohydrate content, it also has very little fiber, a nutrient that helps slow digestion and in turn slows the release of sugar into the blood.	Brown basmati rice has been shown to have the least detrimental effect on blood sugar levels. Another great substitute is quinoa.
High-fructose corn syrup (HFCS)	HFCS is a blend of two sugars, fructose and glucose, which are chemically extracted from corn. Being completely composed of simple sugars, HFCS causes huge spikes in blood sugar. Due to high concentrations of fructose, HFCS does not stimulate the reduction in hunger hormones and the increase in satiety hormones the same way other foods do. Therefore, HFCS is also linked to obesity, which also negatively impacts blood sugar.	There aren't any great substitutes because all sweeteners spike your sugar levels. Instead, focus on bringing out the natural flavors—including sweetness!—in foods with spices and herbs, and such cooking techniques as browning and caramelizing.
Cornstarch	The word starch in its name gives this one away. Cornstarch is purely a carbohydrate, and it has an extremely high glycemic index, which is an indication of how quickly carbohydrates are absorbed into our system and how high the resulting blood sugar spike is. In other words, cornstarch is readily absorbed by our bodies and will spike blood sugars to extremely high levels.	Similarly to HFCS, there is no good substitute. Common substitutes such as flour, potato starch and tapioca will have the same harmful effect on blood sugar levels. Instead, thicken soups and stews with pureed vegetables, and thicken sauces by reducing them (heating them to boil off some of the water) until you obtain the desired thickness.
Juice	Many people believe that juice is a beneficial addition to their diet—it is full of vitamins and minerals! True, but it lacks the other beneficial components of fruits and vegetables (i.e., fiber), which get removed during the juicing process, leaving only the sugar and water. Juice is basically a natural form of a sugar-sweetened beverage, and it will cause your blood sugar to skyrocket. Instead, enjoy whole fruits and vegetables to get the beneficial fiber along with those vitamins and minerals. Note: Juice is beneficial, however, in treating hypoglycemia, or low blood sugar.	Try adding pureed frozen fruit cubes to regular or sparkling water for a hint of sweetness in your drink. Whole frozen pieces of fruit also act as great sweetening ice cubes. If you prefer your water at room temperature, you can add pieces of room temperature fruit. Homemade unsweetened iced tea is also a great option. Simply make your favorite hot tea, let it cool and enjoy!
Bagels	Bagels are sugar spikers for many reasons, the main one being their sheer size. One bagel is equivalent to about 4 slices of bread; that's 4 servings of carbohydrates in one food! In addition, bagels are usually made from refined flours, meaning they lack fiber and other important nutrients.	Sprouted whole-grain English muffins (e.g., Ezekiel 4:9 brand) are a great substitute for bagels. They're doughier than bread, making the consistency more similar to that of a bagel.
Chinese food	Chinese food is a sugar spiker because it contains high amounts of many blood sugar spikers including cornstarch, monosodium glutamate (MSG) and added sugar.	Homemade Chinese food is a much healthier option. Create healthy versions of your favorite sauces, steam some vegetables and enjoy with brown basmati rice or quinoa.

(continued)

SUGAR SPIKER	WHY IT SPIKES SUGARS	GOOD SUBSTITUTES
Sicilian pizza	Sicilian pizza isn't just a regular slice of pizza; it's particularly bad for blood sugar due to its extra-thick crust. A typical slice of Sicilian pizza is the equivalent of 3 or 4 slices of bread, or 45–60 grams of carbs! On top of that, most pizzas are made with white flour, which is refined and does not contain the same filling fiber that whole-grain fiber contains. The lack of fiber means all of those carbohydrates are quickly and easily digested, and go straight into your bloodstream.	Although not the best option, even a slice of regular pizza is better than Sicilian style pizza. The best option would be to either make your own pizza on sprouted whole-grain English muffins (e.g., Ezekiel 4:9 brand) or your own homemade 100% whole grain dough. Whenever eating pizza, always try to squeeze as many veggies as possible on top and add a green salad as well!
Hero/ hoagies/subs	No matter what you call them, these sandwiches are sugar spikers, for sure! Too often, these sandwiches are extra-large and contain more bread than fillings. For a reference, just the bread of a 6-inch (15-cm) Subway sandwich has 5–6 carbohydrate servings!	If you're eating a sandwich, your best option is to make your own on yummy sprouted whole-grain bread (e.g., Ezekiel 4:9 brand). If you are ordering out from a deli or sandwich shop, go for a simple sandwich on two slices of normal, 100% whole-grain bread.
Burritos	Burritos are sugar spikers because they contain too many grams of carbohydrate—tortillas, beans and rice are all carbs. Although beans can be a great source of protein, they also contain carbs.	Choose a burrito bowl option or ask for your burrito without rice. If you're making the burrito at home, ramp up the nutrition and keep blood sugar normalized with sprouted whole-grain tortillas (e.g., Ezekiel 4:9 brand).
Breakfast cereal	Breakfast cereals are different combinations of refined grains. They lack filling nutrients such as fiber. They are also often enriched—meaning nutrients are taken out and then synthetic forms are added back. On top of that, milk is high in sugar, further driving your blood sugar high.	If you are set on cereal for breakfast, eat homemade granola with unsweetened almond milk. Other great breakfast options include tofu scrambles, chia puddings or a healthy smoothie.

FIBER: HOW FIBER HELPS WITH BLOOD SUGAR CONTROL

Fiber digests completely differently than carbohydrates do. Dietary fiber includes all parts of plant foods that our bodies cannot digest or absorb. Fiber does not convert into glucose or add calories to your diet. Therefore it is your best friend for weight loss.

Fiber is classified as soluble or insoluble. Insoluble fiber adds bulk to stools and promotes regular bowel movements. Soluble fiber dissolves in water and can help to lower cholesterol and blood sugar levels. Eating a high-fiber diet can aid in weight loss by filling you up faster and keeping you full longer. It may even reduce your risk of certain forms of cancer!

Here are some food sources of each type of fiber:

Insoluble Fiber	Soluble Fiber
Nuts	Barley
Seeds	Flaxseeds
Vegetables	Legumes
Wheat bran	Oats
Whole wheat flour	Some fruits and vegetables

BEST SOURCES OF FIBER FOR A PLANT-BASED DIET

	Serving Size	Grams of Fiber
Whole Grains		
Barley	½ cup (26 g), uncooked	16
Oats, steelcut	¼ cup (20 g)	5
Sprouted grain bread	1 slice	3
Fruits		
Apples with skin	1 medium	5.00
Avocado	1 medium	11.84
Blueberries	1 cup (148 g)	4.18
Figs, dried	2 medium	3.74
Grapefruit	½ medium	6.12
Orange, navel	1 medium	3.40
Pear	1 medium	5.08
Raspberries	1 cup (123 g)	8.34
Strawberries	1 cup (152 g)	3.98
Vegetables		
Beet greens	1 cup (340 g), cooked	4.20
Bok choy	1 cup (340 g), cooked	2.76
Broccoli	1 cup (230 g), cooked	2.30
Brussels sprouts	1 cup (200 g), cooked	2.84
Cabbage	1 cup (340 g), cooked	4.20
Carrot	1 medium	2.00
Carrot	1 cup (200 g), cooked	5.22
Cauliflower	1 cup (230 g), cooked	3.43
Collard greens	1 cup (340 g), cooked	2.58

(continued)

BEST SOURCES OF FIBER FOR A PLANT-BASED DIET		
	Serving Size	**Grams of Fiber**
Vegetables (continued)		
Onions	1 cup (130 g), raw	2.88
Peas	1 cup (200 g), cooked	8.84
Peppers, sweet	1 cup (170 g)	2.62
Spinach	1 cup (340 g), cooked	4.32
Summer squash	1 cup (200 g), cooked	2.52
Sweet potato	1 cup (200 g), cooked	5.94
Swiss chard	1 cup (340 g), cooked	3.68
Winter squash	1 cup (200 g), cooked	5.74
Nuts and beans		
Almonds	1 ounce (29 g)	4.22
Black beans	1 cup (200 g), cooked	14.92
Flaxseeds	3 tablespoons (30 g)	6.97
Garbanzo beans (chickpeas)	1 cup (200 g), cooked	5.80
Kidney beans	1 cup (200 g), cooked	13.33
Lentils, red	1 cup (200 g), cooked	15.64
Lima beans	1 cup (200 g), cooked	13.16
Pistachio nuts	1 ounce (30 g)	3.10
Pumpkin seeds	¼ cup (40 g)	4.12
Quinoa	½ cup (68 g), uncooked	6 g
Soybeans	1 cup (200 g), cooked	7.62
Sunflower seeds	¼ cup (40 g)	3.00
Walnuts	1 ounce (30 g)	3.08

DAILY FOOD DIARY

It is a good idea to keep a daily food journal. Write down everything you eat and drink—at least for one week. You can also calculate your grams of carbs and net carbs. This will give you great insight into your daily habits and how many carbs you are consuming. Studies show that people who keep food diaries lose the most amount of weight.

MEAL	FOOD EATEN	GRAMS OF CARBS	GRAMS OF FIBER	NET CARBS
Breakfast				
Lunch				
Snack				
Dinner				
Physical activity for the day: Light, Moderate, Vigorous				

YOUR DAILY CARBOHYDRATE MEAL PLAN	
Breakfast	grams of carbs
Lunch	grams of carbs
Snack	grams of carbs
Dinner	grams of carbs

Tips

1. Start to replace all white flours with whole-grain products.

2. When going out to restaurants, ask your server to omit the "carbs," such as rice or mashed potatoes, and replace with vegetables.

3. Eat more fruits and vegetables. Aim for two servings of vegetables at lunch and dinner and two or three pieces of fruit every day.

4. Eat more beans and legumes. Try adding these to soups or salads.

5. Start to make your lunches and bring to work instead of buying lunch.

To-Do List

❑ Cut out all white and refined products.

❑ Look at labels for grams of carbohydrate and start counting your carbs.

❑ Start to keep daily food and carbohydrate journal.

❑ Gradually increase the fiber in your diet until you are up to 25 to 35 grams per day, by the end of the week.

JOSIE'S STORY
I went down two dress sizes and was finally able to get my blood sugar under control.

I have had type 1 diabetes since I was 6 years old. I am 36 now. I have always struggled with the highs and lows that come along with trying to manage insulin dependent diabetes. It has never been easy for me. I have had many complications that come along with diabetes, like tingling in my fingers and toes, and I have been hospitalized twice in the past few years because I became unconscious due to a low blood sugar. I couldn't take the ups and the downs anymore—I didn't know what to do. I was desperate. I went to see my doctor and he sent me to Cher.

The first thing she did was say that I needed to change the way I had been eating. I knew that I had to make changes, but before seeing her I didn't know where to start. She gave me the knowledge and inspiration to begin, and she recommended I start following this diet. I am from the Dominican Republic, so I was used to eating a lot of fried food, white rice and very little vegetables. I also love sweets and steak!

I cut out all fried foods and animal products and the sweets, too. She told me not to buy any fake products or fat-free things because they contain more sugar, high-fructose corn syrup and sugar alcohols. For the first time ever I started to buy real food—fresh fruits and vegetables, and whole grains. Before I started following this way of eating, I never ate any vegetables—it just wasn't a part of my diet. I would eat a lot of rice and processed carbs, and I would snack on anything sweet I could get my hands on. I would have French fries and donuts whenever I wanted. All the while, not making the connection between what I was eating and how it was affecting my blood sugar. I was trying to manage my diet and blood sugar, but it always seemed out of my reach. Not only was my blood sugar poorly controlled, but I was also the fattest I had ever been in my life.

In the beginning of the 28-day meal plan, I didn't know how I was going to make it. How could I give up sweets or animal products? But I committed to the 28 days, and I said I would do it. Halfway through the 28 days, I was already feeling better, and I was losing weight. My cravings decreased, my energy went up and I was taking half the amount of insulin that I was taking before. It was so inspiring that I was eager to continue. Now here I am 6 months later, and I have lost 20 pounds (9 kg), I am feeling much better and I could never imagine not eating this way. My mood is better because I don't have the rapidly fluctuating blood sugars, and I am much more stable. I am so grateful that I found Cher and that I changed my way of eating. It truly saved my life.

CHAPTER 3

ZERO DIABETES

Americans are sicker and less healthy than other people in wealthy, developed nations. Can you believe that? That is appalling! It is due in large part to what we are eating and the amount of exercise that we are getting.

But don't be dismayed! You can change it. You don't have to be sick. You don't have to be overweight. You don't have to get diabetes! You have much more control than you think. It starts with making a commitment to yourself. A commitment to eat healthy and nutritious foods and to be more physically active. I will show you how to do it—all you have to do is start following the principles of the BSM and watch your life transform. You will start to feel better, lower your blood sugar, have more energy and see the weight disappear.

THE SIX PRINCIPLES OF
THE BLOOD SUGAR MIRACLE (BSM)

1. Avoid Highly Processed Foods

People are consuming the greatest quantity of processed foods now more than in any other time in history. However, most people don't even know how dangerous these foods are. Recent studies show that processed foods are linked to many common diseases, including diabetes, heart disease, certain cancers and obesity. Can you believe so many diseases can come from the foods you eat? Does anyone else find this alarming? Am I the only one? Well, what are we going to do about it? First, we need to know what the highly processed foods are, and then we need to change the way we eat.

What exactly is processed food? Processed food is anything that has been altered from its original form. The degree to which it has been altered appears to be the bigger problem. The processed foods that I am talking about here are the ones that come in a bag, box, jar, package or can with a list of ingredients a mile long—sometimes called ultraprocessed food. Some examples of common processed foods include white flour, artificial sweeteners, cakes, cookies, pastries, breakfast cereals, soft drinks, sugary "fruit" drinks, cheese food, frozen dinners, processed meat products (sausage, bologna, bacon, packaged ham, etc.) and refined sugars (including high-fructose corn syrup). Most processed foods are stripped of all nutrients and are high in sugar, fat, salt and calories.

Processed foods were created for several reasons, including to improve shelf life, preserve, texturize, soften and sweeten. It is no coincidence that processed foods are also convenience foods and are quick and easy to consume. Data shows that about 90 percent of the food we eat today is processed. Part of the problem is that the more processed a food is, the easier it is for the body to break it down—meaning that it will turn into sugar faster and be stored as fat instead of being used for energy. In addition, processed foods are not whole or natural—which is an essential principle of the BSM way.

Here are some of the worst ingredients in processed foods and why they are bad for you:

INGREDIENT	WHY IT'S BAD FOR YOU
High-fructose corn syrup (HFCS)	Consuming HFCS leads to obesity and other diseases, such as diabetes. Since HFCS is not natural and has been genetically modified, no digestion is required, and it enters your bloodstream more rapidly. Because it enters your bloodstream as fructose, it triggers the production of fats, such as cholesterol and triglycerides. If your cholesterol and triglycerides remain high, you are at risk for fatty liver and heart disease. In addition, HFCS is found in overly processed foods; it does not occur in whole, natural foods, which is another reason to avoid it.
Artificial sweeteners	The main problems with artificial sweeteners are that they enhance your appetite for sweet things and contribute to greater weight gain than sugar does. And they alter the flora in the gut; new studies are showing that this also contributes to weight gain. If it isn't yet clear, weight gain leads to many diseases, including heart disease and diabetes.
Monosodium glutamate (MSG)	MSG is found in countless processed food products. The biggest problem with MSG is that it overstimulates the nervous system, which then causes an inflammatory response; inflammation in the body leads to many diseases.
Refined/enriched flour	The biggest problem with refined and enriched food products is that many of the nutrients have been stripped away (and later added back in), and the fiber has been removed as well. These products break down faster, leading to a spike in blood sugar because they enter the bloodstream rapidly.
Preservatives	Many preservatives are linked to a host of health problems, including hyperactivity, certain kinds of cancer and possible allergic reactions.
Artificial colors	Artificial coloring in foods is linked to many health issues, including cancer, hyperactivity and allergy-like reactions.

Not only are highly processed foods bad, but sugar, in particular added sugar, is really bad for you. With the food industry using a variety of names to mask sugar as an ingredient, it is no wonder why we are confused and sick. Take a look at the following table to find all the other names of sugar used in highly processed foods.

OTHER NAMES FOR SUGAR	
Agave nectar	Produced from several species of agave
Barley malt syrup	A natural, unrefined sweetener produced from sprouted malted barley. Composed of about 65% maltose, 30% complex carbohydrate and 3% protein
Brown rice syrup	Brown rice syrup comes from (you guessed it!) brown rice. More nutritious than its high-fructose alternative, this buttery and nutty-flavored syrup is commonly found in granola bars and baked breads
Brown sugar	Brown table sugar (sucrose) and molasses
Cane sugar	Processed sugarcane
Cane syrup	Processed sugarcane
Coconut palm sugar	Natural sweetener from coconut palm trees. Made by tapping the sweet nectar from the tropical coconut palm tree flower and drying the juice in a large, open kettle drum. Contains potassium
Confectioners' sugar	Also known as powdered sugar. It is plain white granulated sugar, but processed to a superfine consistency
Corn sweetener	See "corn syrup"
Corn syrup	Made from cornstarch. Corn syrup is used in foods to soften texture, add volume, prevent crystallization of sugar and enhance flavor. Not the same as HFCS
Date sugar	Made from dehydrated, ground dates
Dextrose	Another name for glucose
Fructose	Sugar that occurs naturally in fruits, vegetables and honey
Fruit juice concentrate	Made when water is removed from whole juice to make it more concentrated
Glucose	Simple sugar, our main source of energy. Circulates in the bloodstream
Granulated white sugar	Table sugar. Made by processing raw sugar from sugarcane or sugar beets
High-fructose corn syrup	A combination of fructose and glucose, made by processing corn syrup
Honey	A mix of glucose, fructose and sucrose created from nectar collected by bees
Invert sugar	A mix of fructose and glucose made by processing sucrose. Used as a preservative
Inverted cane syrup	Sucrose split into a mixture of glucose and fructose

OTHER NAMES FOR SUGAR	
Lactose	Occurs naturally in milk
Malt syrup	Made from evaporated corn mash and sprouted barley. Also known as malt sugar
Maltose	Starch and malt broken down into simple sugars and used commonly in beer, bread and baby food
Maple syrup	Made from the sap of the maple tree
Molasses	The thick, dark syrup that's left after sugar beets or sugarcane is processed for table sugar
Palm sugar	See "coconut palm sugar"
Raw sugar	The product of the first stage of the cane sugar refining process
Refined white sugar	See "table sugar"
Sorghum syrup	Made from juice extracted from sorghum cane
Sucrose	Table sugar
Sugar alcohols	Extracted from plants or manufactured from sugars and starches. Not completely absorbed by the body. Different ones affect the gastrointestinal tract differently
Erythritol	A sugar alcohol that is 60% to 70% as sweet as sugar
Isomalt	A sugar alcohol that has a small effect on blood sugar; can cause GI distress
Lactitol	A sugar alcohol that is about 40% as sweet as sugar. It is also used as a laxative
Maltitol	A sugar alcohol that is 70% to 90% sweeter than sugar
Mannitol	A sugar alcohol that also acts as a diuretic
Sorbitol	A sugar alcohol that is slowly metabolized. Most sorbitol is made from corn syrup
Xylitol	A sugar alcohol that is 33% sweeter than sugar
Sugarcane juice	Juice extracted from pressured sugarcane
Table sugar	Sucrose (granulated white sugar)
Turbinado syrup	Sucrose split into a mixture of glucose and fructose
White sugar	Table sugar (granulated white sugar)
Whole cane sugar	Made from whole, unrefined, evaporated sugarcane juice

2. Avoid Red Meat and Most Animal Products

In addition to avoiding highly processed foods, eating fewer animal products will have a huge impact on your health. Eating fewer animal products is the key to preventing chronic diseases including obesity, heart disease and type 2 diabetes, because animal products are high in saturated fat and cholesterol and are often polluted by hormones and antibiotics. The biggest problems with animal products in this country are how they are produced and that we are consuming too much of them. The consumption of animal products has almost doubled during the last few decades. Increased health issues in our society is a direct result. Start to eat fewer animal products, and your health will dramatically improve.

Studies have shown that a small increase in red meat can increase your risk of type 2 diabetes. If you decrease your consumption of animal protein, you will reduce your risk of getting diabetes.

The problem with red meat:

WHAT'S THE BEEF?	WHY BEEF IS BAD
GMOs	Most cows are fed corn from genetically modified crops.
Growth hormones	Cattle are pumped full of growth hormones.
Undesirable fats	Beef contains higher amounts of saturated fat and omega-6 fatty acids and less omega-3 fatty acids
Obesogens	Obesogens are chemicals that have been found to disrupt the endocrine system and promote weight gain and obesity.
Antibiotics	Antibiotics are given to livestock to make them plump. They will make you plump as well.

3. Eat Whole Natural Foods

Eating a whole foods diet means maximizing your nutrient intake and obtaining your foods from natural sources while avoiding the highly processed foods. Whole natural foods include fruits, vegetables, nuts and seeds, legumes and whole grains. A whole food is a food that is as close to its natural state as possible, such as a stalk of broccoli, a raw almond or a scoop of quinoa. As opposed to potato chips, fruit juice or a candy bar.

Understanding nutrient density is important—nutrient density essentially means the amount of nutrients in a food given the number of calories it contains. Nutrient-dense foods give you the most amount of nutrients for the least amount of calories. Nutrient-dense foods help you lose weight and fight off diseases because you can eat a lot of them and get full on fewer calories. No foods are more nutrient dense than whole and natural foods.

When you consume more whole foods, the amount of highly processed foods you eat will naturally and easily fall by the wayside. Choose whole foods as often as possible while avoiding such foods as white bread, crackers, chips, candies and cookies.

4. Eat Your Fruits and Vegetables

It may sound clichéd and kind of boring, but it is true and very important. The fact that it has to be mentioned is the real problem. The typical American diet today includes very few vegetables. Vegetables are a great source of vitamins and minerals, antioxidants, water and fiber—all of which are important for your body to function optimally. In addition, they are low in calories, so they are your best friend when you are trying to lose weight. Most vegetables can be eaten in abundance. Some, however, you have to count as a "carb;" for example, starchier vegetables include corn, peas, potatoes, beets and some squashes, such as acorn and butternut. While these vegetables are nutritious, you do have to monitor the quantity consumed for optimal blood sugar control (see Chapter 2). Once you start to increase your vegetable and fruit intake, your desire for animal products and junk food will decline, and you will automatically feel healthier.

Studies show that people who eat more fruits and vegetables daily dramatically reduce their risk of getting type 2 diabetes.

FIVE TIPS TO INCREASE YOUR VEGETABLE AND FRUIT INTAKE

1. You have to buy them! It may sound obvious, but if you aren't used to eating them, you will have to make it a point to include them in your weekly shopping list. Once you have them at home, prepare them quickly. For example, cut up fresh veggies and put them in containers, so when you come home hungry from work, you can grab them. Cook a big batch of vegetable soup, so you have it ready for those late nights. Rinse your lettuce, spin it dry and then cut it up into pieces, so it will be ready to make a salad at any minute.

2. Wash your fruit as soon as you get it home from the market. If you have it all washed and ready to eat, you will be much more likely to reach for it. In fact you can do a little test. If you are home and feel hungry, ask yourself whether you want to eat an apple (or another whole fruit). If the answer is yes, then you are hungry. If the answer is no, then you are likely not hungry, and you are looking to fill another emotion (maybe you are bored or tired). Try it—it works!

3. Keep it exciting! Make one new vegetable dish each week. Most people say they don't like vegetables, but the reality is most people haven't tried that many veggies. And if they have tried them, the veggies were likely prepared in a really boring and tasteless way. Often vegetables are steamed or overcooked, leaving them not tasting so great. It doesn't have to be like that! Try quickly sautéing spinach in a bit of extra-virgin olive oil with garlic. You can even make it spicy by adding red pepper flakes—yum! There are many more delicious vegetable recipes in this book (see Chapter 11).

4. Think of vegetables as the main attraction on your plate instead of as the side dish. Maybe when you were growing up, vegetables were not the main attraction—or they may not have even made it onto your plate! If this is a little out of your comfort zone, make the transition gradually, and you will never know a time when you didn't eat your veggies.

5. It is easy to increase the fruit in your diet. Make it your go-to snack, blend it in a smoothie or bake it for a healthy dessert.

5. Control Your Carbohydrate Intake

We talked about carbohydrates in depth in Chapter 2, so what I will say here is try to limit carbohydrates to no more than 30 grams in one meal for women and 45 grams for men, while keeping your dietary fiber intake between 30 and 50 grams per day.

6. Exercise, Exercise, Exercise!

Being physically active is one of the most important things you can do for your body. Our society has evolved into one where if you didn't go out of your way to do it, you wouldn't have any physical activity at all. You could wake up, drive to work, sit at your desk all day, eat lunch at your desk, go home, eat dinner, watch television and go to sleep. Does that sound familiar? This is a big problem facing our society. This type of living is what leads to obesity, high blood pressure, prediabetes and potentially, type 2 diabetes. It really must change. Society as a whole has to change. You need to make physical activity part of your daily routine. Perhaps you can bike or walk to work. Or maybe you can get out for 30 minutes to take a walk at lunch. If you can't find a way to build it into your daily life, then you will need to find another outlet. Do you remember how active you were when you were a little kid? You probably couldn't sit still for very long! You couldn't wait to get outside and play. You need to think like that again. Maybe you can join some kind of sports team, such as basketball or volleyball, or join a walking or running club in your community. It is a great way to meet new people and become physically active. Join a gym, try a new exercise class, buy a hula hoop, get some exercise videos, try gardening or buy a bike! Another great way to increase your exercise is to get an activity tracker; for example, a Fitbit or a Nike FuelBand. Think of any way you can move more and be physically active in your daily life.

The benefits of exercise are innumerable. Exercise is the key to maintaining a healthy weight: It will help you ward off many diseases, it will help you manage your stress and clear your mind and it will significantly help you lower your blood sugar.

EXERCISE AND TYPE 2 DIABETES

Physical activity is a key factor in the prevention and management of type 2 diabetes. "Exercise plays a major role in the prevention and control of insulin resistance, prediabetes, GDM (gestational diabetes), type 2 diabetes and diabetes-related health complications. Both aerobic and resistance training improve insulin action, at least acutely, and can assist with the management of blood glucose levels, lipids, blood pressure, cardiovascular risk, mortality and quality of life, but exercise must be undertaken regularly to have continued benefits and likely include regular training of varying types."[17]

According to the American College of Sports Medicine (ACSM) and the ADA clinical practice recommendation and statements, here are some of the benefits of exercise on type 2 diabetes:

1. Physical activity can result in bodywide improvements in insulin action and can last from 2 to 72 hours.
2. Both aerobic and resistance training improve insulin action, blood glucose control and fat oxidation and storage in muscle.
3. Increased physical activity can reduce symptoms of depression and improve quality of life in people with type 2 diabetes.
4. At least 2½ hours per week of moderate to vigorous exercise should be undertaken to prevent type 2 diabetes in high-risk individuals.
5. Studies suggest that physical activity may reduce the risk of developing gestational diabetes during pregnancy.

6. It is recommended that people with type 2 diabetes get 150 minutes per week of physical activity. It should be spread out over three days of the week and no more than two consecutive days without physical activity.

So, get moving! (Consult with your doctor before starting any exercise routine.)

A Few Words about Protein

Protein is an important component of your daily food intake. Like carbs and fat, protein is found in almost every part of your body and, just like carbs and fat, you don't want to consume too much. For decades we have been encouraged to eat way too much protein—and it continues to increase. The main problem with that is that the biggest sources of protein in the typical American diet come from meats, cheese and dairy.

How do you know how much you should have? A basic amount of protein recommended for a healthy adult is 0.8 grams per kilogram of body weight. So, for a 150-pound (68 kg) person, that is about 55 grams per day. This amount would vary depending on age, athletic needs and illnesses, including hypermetabolic states and kidney disease.

Protein has minimal effect on blood sugar levels; however, recent research has shown high-protein diets may contribute to glucose disturbances. Additionally, when carbohydrates are eaten with a protein or a fat (or fiber), it slows down how quickly the glucose is converted to blood sugars, which lessens the amount of insulin needed to combat the increase in blood sugar. This is why it is important to eat a balance of carbs, protein and good fats (fatty acids) on a daily basis.

Recent studies show that a high-protein diet is associated with several diseases, including cardiovascular disease, some cancers and type 2 diabetes. In the past several years, a high-protein, extremely low-carb diet (e.g., the Atkins diet) has shown favorable results on body weight and glucose homeostasis in short-term interventions. But, "In contrast, a cross-sectional study related long-term high protein intake to elevated glucose concentrations and insulin resistance in healthy individuals."[18] Just as when we talked about carbs in Chapter 2, you want to know how much protein to get and then get it from the best sources.

In a plant-based diet, many people are concerned with getting enough protein. But if you plan it properly, a plant-based diet can give you the recommended amount of protein to help you maintain a healthy weight and ward off diabetes. Great sources of plant protein include beans (including soybeans), tofu, tempeh, nuts, seeds and green leafy vegetables.

THE BEST PLANT-BASED PROTEIN SOURCES

Food Source	Serving Size	Total Protein
Tempeh	½ package	20 g
Lentils	1 cup (200 g), cooked	18 g
Beans	1 cup (200 g), cooked	14.5 g
Hemp seeds	3 tablespoons (30 g)	10 g
Quinoa	1 cup (160 g), cooked	9 g
Tofu	3 ounces (85 g)	9 g
Sunflower seeds	4 tablespoons (40 g)	8 g
Food Source	Serving Size	Total Protein
Broccoli	1 cup (230 g)	7 g
Chia seeds	2 tablespoons (20 g)	6 g
Edamame	½ cup (100 g), cooked	6 g

A Few Words about Alcohol

If you don't already drink, then don't start drinking! However, most people with type 2 diabetes can safely have alcohol in moderation. For women that means one alcoholic drink per day; and for men it is two. A drink equals 12 ounces (340 ml) of beer, 5 ounces (140 ml) of wine or 1.5 ounces (42 ml) of distilled spirits.

But before you take that drink, wait! While alcohol may be safe in moderation, if you are trying to prevent diabetes, reverse a type 2 diagnosis or lose weight, alcohol will hinder your progress. Alcohol packs a double-whammy punch. (1) Alcohol contains empty calories. There are no nutrients in alcohol that your body can use, so it is just wasted calories. (2) Alcohol decreases your body's ability to metabolize fat. So, you have calories that head straight to your fat stores, and your body will only be burning fat at half the rate that it should.

If you are taking any medication, you shouldn't drink alcohol, as it can interfere with most medications. Also, if you are on insulin, you shouldn't drink alcohol. And in all cases, you should check with your doctor before consuming alcohol.

A Few Words about Caffeine

Caffeine appears safe for healthy people in the amount of about 400 milligrams per day or about two 8-ounce (237 ml) cups of coffee (equal to one Starbucks Grande regular coffee). In fact, some recent studies have shown that caffeine may reduce your risk of developing type 2 diabetes. However, if you already have type 1 or type 2 diabetes, you may want to reconsider drinking caffeine, as the impact of caffeine may be associated with higher or lower blood sugar levels.

A Few Words about Organic Foods

"Organic farming uses an approach to growing crops and raising livestock that avoids synthetic chemicals, hormones, antibiotic agents, genetic engineering and irradiation."[19] Buy organic if you can and it fits into your budget.

Take care to distinguish between the following food marketing terms:

COMMONLY USED FOOD PRODUCT MARKETING TERMS	
100% organic	Must contain only organically produced ingredients and processing aids (excluding water and salt)
Organic	Must consist of at least 95% organically produced ingredients (excluding salt and water). Any remaining product ingredients must consist of nonagricultural substances approved on the national list.
Made with organic ingredients	Must contain at least 70% organic ingredients
Natural	A product containing no artificial ingredient or added color and that is only minimally processed (a process that does not fundamentally alter the raw product). The label must explain the use of the term.

A Few Words about GMOs

Genetically modified organisms, or GMOs, are plants or animals that have been genetically altered in a laboratory through genetic engineering. These products do not exist naturally in nature. GMOs are designed to have increased crop yield and are a strong defense against pests and drought issues. However, GMOs have been linked to health problems, including allergies, disturbances in the reproductive cycle and certain cancers.

Examples of GMOs include soybeans, corn, and canola and cottonseed oil.

Read food packaging carefully to find soy and other healthy products that carry the "non-GMO" verified seal. Avoid genetically modified foods.

Tips

1. Start to think of plants as you would meat. Build your meal around the plant and not the meat.
2. Bring your lunch to work. It will save you money as well as reduce your waistline.
3. Don't buy highly processed foods. If you don't have them in the house, you won't eat them.
4. Start your day with a morning walk.
5. Buy more whole foods and produce and less red meat, and you will greatly reduce your intake of sugar and saturated fat.

To-Do List

❑ Stack your shopping cart with fruits and vegetables this week.

❑ Fill half of your lunch and dinner plate with vegetables.

❑ Start walking and make an appointment with your doctor to get cleared to exercise.

❑ Consider purchasing an activity tracker.

CHAPTER 4

MICRONUTRIENTS— YOUR NEW BEST FRIENDS

There are several key micronutrients that help reduce your type 2 diabetes risk as well as keep your essential nutrient requirements at an optimum level. Since the BSM plan is all about whole foods (versus easy supplements), it should be of no surprise that the best sources of these micronutrients are found in real food! However, in some cases, supplements may be necessary. As with any nutrition plan, if you are on any type of prescribed medicine, please consult your physician before supplementing your diet with any vitamins or minerals, as some may have an adverse reaction to certain medications.

MAGNESIUM

Why It's Good

Magnesium, the fourth-most-abundant mineral in your body, is essential to daily function—yet an estimated 80 percent of Americans are magnesium deficient. Magnesium is key to 300 different chemical reactions in the body, including sustaining the health of your heart and blood vessels, maintaining your energy level and helping you relax. If you are attuned to famous ad campaigns, then you'll remember the famous milk of magnesia ads over the years. Yes, magnesium does help alleviate constipation. In addition to calcium, magnesium is also essential for bone health. Doctors prescribe it as a blood thinner as well. Last, and most important, magnesium has been shown to be key for diabetes prevention. Magnesium helps glucose enter the cells. So, if you want to optimize your metabolism and reduce your risk for type 2 diabetes, you need to consume adequate magnesium.

Latest Research on How It Helps Diabetes Prevention

Elevated insulin has been linked to low magnesium levels in recent studies. People with insulin resistance experience increased excretion of magnesium in their urine, as well as increased urinary glucose. This contributes to diminished magnesium levels and increased urinary output. As such, the lower your magnesium levels, the less your body is able to retain it.

A 2013 ADA study revealed that higher magnesium intake reduces risk of impaired glucose and insulin metabolism and slows progression from prediabetes to diabetes, especially in middle-aged Americans.[20] Scientists say that a deficiency of magnesium interrupts insulin secretion in the pancreas and increases insulin resistance in the body's tissues, resulting in a decrease in blood sugar control in type 2 diabetes. A recent analysis also showed that people with higher dietary intakes of magnesium (through consumption of whole grains, nuts and green leafy vegetables) had a decreased risk of type 2 diabetes.

Men should consume 420 mg per day and women should consume 320 mg.

Best Sources of Magnesium

FOOD SOURCE	SERVING SIZE	TOTAL MAGNESIUM
Squash/pumpkin seeds	½ cup (80 g)	606 mg
Brazil nuts	½ cup (75 g)	252 mg
Almonds	½ cup (85 g)	192 mg
Cashews	½ cup (55 g)	176 mg
Spinach	1 cup (340 g), raw	157 mg
Swiss chard	1 cup (180 g)	152 mg
Soybeans	1 cup (200 g), cooked	148 mg
Peanuts	½ cup (75 g)	124 mg
Quinoa	1 cup (160 g), cooked	120 mg

(continued)

FOOD SOURCE	SERVING SIZE	TOTAL MAGNESIUM
French beans	1 cup (200 g)	100 mg
Dark chocolate	1 square	95 mg
Black-eyed peas	1 cup (150 g), cooked	92 mg
Kidney beans	1 cup (200 g), cooked	86 mg
Brown rice	1 cup (210 g), cooked	86 mg
Garbanzo beans (chickpeas)	1 cup (200 g), cooked	80 mg

TIM'S STORY:
I'm not obese anymore!

I have been overweight my whole life. But it was never this bad. In fact, before I started working with Cher, my weight was so high that I couldn't even check it on the scale at the doctor's office. One scale went up to 350 pounds (158.6 kg) and the other one went up to 440 pounds (199.6 kg). My weight didn't register. It was devastating.

In high school and college I was always "big"—bigger than most of my friends. But I was active, and I played football and I managed it. But 20 years later and after sitting at a computer all day, I had gained over 200 pounds (90 kg). It wasn't manageable anymore. The only good news was that at least I was "healthy." I didn't (yet) have any of the diseases that go along with being 200 pounds (90 kg) overweight. I didn't have high blood pressure, my cholesterol was fine and I wasn't diabetic. Thankfully. But I knew I had to do something or else that would be my future.

I first started with moving more. I started walking. In the beginning I couldn't do that much, but within no time I was walking 2 miles per day—I did this Monday through Friday. Then I started walking on the weekends for longer than 2 miles. It felt good. I could see that I was getting stronger, and I was starting to feel better.

Then Cher and I started to change the way I had been eating. I started slowly. First, I had to cut out all soda. I did. It wasn't that hard. Then I started to cut down on the "carbs"—especially the ones that were really bad for me, like cakes and cookies and candies. It took me a little while to get these out of my life, but I stuck with it and I did it. Now I don't really even want them anymore. I still eat rice, but now I eat brown rice and I have 1½ cups (315 g) instead of 3 cups (630 g). And I always have a vegetable on the side. I am drinking 80 ounces (2.2 L) of water per day. I am taking my vitamin D$_3$ every day. I am walking every day. Then, I started to cut down on animal products. I first gave up dairy—again, not that hard. And once I saw the weight starting to come off, it made it much easier to keep going. I have now given up all animal products, and I have lost 90 pounds (40 kg) over the past year. I still have a ways to go, but I am doing it, and I know I will get there. I am so grateful that I started eating like this and that I changed my life.

CHROMIUM

Why It's Good

Chromium is a metallic element that we require in minute amounts, yet it is an essential part of metabolic processes that helps insulin transport glucose into cells, where it can be used for energy—as well as regulate blood sugar. Chromium is also involved in the metabolism of carbohydrate, fat and protein. Chromium can also help prevent heart disease and raise HDL ("good") cholesterol levels.

Latest Research on How It Helps Diabetes Prevention

Chromium is needed to make glucose tolerance factor (GTF), which helps improve insulin action. Inadequate intake of chromium has been linked to the development of glucose intolerance, which is evident in type 2 diabetes.

Best Sources of Chromium

While the best sources should be obtained from food, two forms of supplements are commonly available—glucose-tolerance factor chromium and chromium picolinate. Some medications can alter stomach acidity and may reduce chromium absorption or increase excretion of chromium; if you are on medications, please consult your registered dietician or physician before taking any supplements.

I recommend between 200 and 800 mcg (micrograms) of chromium per day for both men and women.

FOOD SOURCE	SERVING SIZE	TOTAL CHROMIUM
Shredded wheat	1 ounce (29 g)	33 mcg
Peas	½ cup (75 g)	30 mcg
Broccoli	½ cup (115 g)	11 mcg
Grape juice	1 cup (237 g)	8 mcg
Whole wheat English muffin	1 muffin	4 mcg
Potatoes	1 cup (200 g)	3 mcg
Garlic	1 teaspoon (4 g)	3 mcg
Basil	1 tablespoon (3 g)	2 mcg
Whole wheat bread	2 slices	2 mcg
Red wine	5 ounces (142 ml)	Variable, 1–13 mcg
Green beans	1 cup (270 g)	2 mcg
Bananas	1 medium	1 mcg
Apples	1 medium	1 mcg
Asparagus	½ cup (25 g)	Variable*
Prunes	5 prunes	Variable*
Mushrooms	1 cup (60 g)	Variable*

*Chromium content varies based on soil content.

BIOTIN

Why It's Good

Biotin, also known as vitamin B$_7$, helps support adrenal function, maintain a healthy nervous system and is a necessary function in fatty acid metabolism and in the production of glucose, of which the last two are also both essential to staying fit. Biotin is also used to treat such conditions as alopecia, cancer, Crohn's disease, hair loss, Parkinson's disease and diabetic neuropathy, for starters.

Latest Research on How It Helps Diabetes Prevention

A study published in the January 2011 issue of *Molecular Genetics and Metabolism* found that biotin deficiency impairs glucose and cholesterol regulation. Researchers also noted that insulin control and production of fats were negatively impacted and glucose production and fatty acid oxidation were increased. Biotin may also decrease insulin resistance.

I recommend 1,000 mcg per day for both men and women.

Best Sources of Biotin

FOOD SOURCE	SERVING SIZE	TOTAL BIOTIN
Peanuts	¼ cup (38 g)	26.28 mcg
Almonds	¼ cup (43 g)	14.72 mcg
Swiss chard	1 cup (180 g)	10.5 mcg
Sweet potato	1 medium	8.6 mcg
Oats	¼ cup (20 g)	7.8 mcg
Tomatoes	1 cup (160 g)	7.2 mcg
Carrots	1 cup (270 g)	6.1 mcg
Walnuts	¼ cup (30 g)	5.7 mcg
Bananas	1 medium	3.07 mcg
Raspberries	1 cup (123 g)	2.34 mcg
Romaine lettuce	2 cups (680 g)	1.79 mcg
Cauliflower	1 cup (230 g)	1.61 mcg
Strawberries	1 cup (151 g)	1.58 mcg
Watermelon	1 cup (160 g)	1.52 mcg
Grapefruit	½ medium	1.28 mcg

VITAMIN B$_{12}$

Why It's Good

Vitamin B$_{12}$, also called cobalamin, is a water-soluble vitamin with a key role in the normal functioning of the brain and nervous system and for the formation of blood. It is one of the eight B vitamins. It is normally involved in the metabolism of every cell of the human body, especially affecting DNA synthesis and regulation, but also fatty acid metabolism and amino acid metabolism.

Latest Research on How It Helps Diabetes Prevention

Vitamin B$_{12}$ is necessary for formation and growth of red blood cells, neurological function, DNA synthesis and to support the digestive system in keeping glucose levels stable. Vitamin B$_{12}$ also helps to build your immune system. Red blood cells attach themselves to oxygen, which they carry along to your tissues. Red blood cells are vitally important. They only live for three short months. So, it's vital that you replenish them. Deficiencies can lead to anemia, fatigue, weakness, constipation, loss of appetite, depression, confusion and dementia. If a B$_{12}$ deficiency is not remedied, permanent nerve damage can occur.

Vitamin B$_{12}$ deficiency is common in those with type 2 diabetes, especially those who are being treated with metformin, a medication that lowers serum vitamin B$_{12}$ levels.[21]

As such B$_{12}$ supplementation is necessary for type 2 diabetics, as well as for those on vegetarian (meatless) diets, since B$_{12}$ comes primarily from animal products.

I recommend supplementing with 50 to 100 mcg of vitamin B$_{12}$ per day for both men and women. In addition, B$_{12}$ levels can be monitored through a simple blood test at your doctor's office. Thus, you can check your levels and adjust your dose accordingly.

Best Sources of Vitamin B$_{12}$

The only reliable source of B$_{12}$ for the BSM plan is a B$_{12}$ supplement, as B$_{12}$ is found only in animal sources. Supplementation can be taken orally or, if the body is unable to absorb B$_{12}$ due to medications or other medical complications, by injection.

VITAMIN D

Why It's Good

As most of you probably know, vitamin D is important for building bones, but it is also essential for other functions in the body, including cardiovascular health and the regulation of metabolism. Vitamin D deficiency is linked to conditions such as certain types of cancer, heart disease, weight gain and depression. For those who live in climates where clouds and rain prevail over sun or those who live in climates that experience traditional fall and winter, seasonal affective disorder (SAD) can also occur due to the lack of vitamin D from the sun. SAD is a form of depression due to the reduced sunlight hours.

Vitamin D is not found in that many foods, and many people today have some form of vitamin D deficiency, which makes it even more important to consume foods rich in this nutrient. As most of us know, the sun is a great source (vitamin D is produced when ultraviolet rays from the sun strike the skin), but it is also found in whole foods.

Latest Research on How It Helps Diabetes Prevention

Research shows that vitamin D levels were more closely linked to blood sugar levels than body mass index (BMI), and people with higher vitamin D levels have a decreased risk of developing type 2 diabetes compared to people with the lower levels.[22]

The study suggests that vitamin D deficiency and obesity may work together to heighten the risk of diabetes. As the deficiency worsened, so did blood sugar control. You may be able to reduce your risk by maintaining a healthy diet and getting enough outdoor activity and sun exposure.

I recommend 1,000 IUs (International Units) of vitamin D per day for both men and women. Again, your vitamin D levels can be checked through a simple blood test at your doctor's office and you can adjust your intake accordingly.

Best Sources of Vitamin D

FOOD	SERVING	VITAMIN D
Portobello mushrooms	1 cup (60 g)	400 IU
Fortified unsweetened soy milk	8 ounces (227 g)	150 IU
Fortified orange juice	8 ounces (227 g)	137 IU
Fortified unsweetened multigrain cereal, (e.g., Cheerios)	1 cup (22 g)	90 IU
Fortified vegan margarine	1 tablespoon (15 g)	60 IU
Shiitake mushrooms	1 cup (60 g)	45 IU
White mushrooms	1 cup (60 g)	5 IU
Sunlight (20–25 minutes per day)		Varies
UV lamp (20–25 minutes per day)		Varies

FOLATE

Why It's Good

Folate, known also as folic acid or vitamin B_9, and taken most commonly by pregnant women (or women in prepregnancy mode), is widely recognized to help prevent birth defects. However, it has health benefits for people of all ages. Folate works with vitamin B_{12} and vitamin C to help the body break down, use and make new proteins. It also helps form red blood cells and produce DNA, the building block of the human body.

Latest Research on How It Helps with Diabetes Prevention

Studies have also shown that folate may help prevent type 2 diabetes, heart disease, depression, Alzheimer's disease and even some forms of cancer. Type 2 diabetes is linked to high levels of fat, triglycerides in particular. Folate may help with the breakdown of triglycerides, which are in the blood and are used for energy. A study by the *European Journal of Endocrinology* also found that women with a BMI of 30 and above also had low levels of folate.[23] Researchers have also documented that folate supplementation (in the form of folic acid) "may have a potential role, especially as primary prevention, in decreasing cardiovascular events in type 2 diabetic patients."[24]

The recommended amount of folate is 400 mcg for both men and women (except pregnant women—then it can be 400, 600, 800 or 1,000 mcg).

Best Sources of Folate

Folate can be found naturally in plenty of food sources, and folic acid is the synthetic form of this vitamin. For the most benefits, try to obtain folate through food rather than in a supplement form.

FOOD	SERVING	TOTAL FOLATE
All-bran cereal, (e.g., Kellogg's All Bran Buds)	⅓ cup (18 g)	1,806 mcg
Spinach	1 cup (180 g)	1,687 mcg
Endive	1 head	1,670 mcg
Romaine lettuce	1 cup (340 g)	1,600 mcg
Asparagus	1 cup (50 g)	1,592 mcg
Mustard greens	1 cup (180 g)	1,445 mcg
Epazote	1 tablespoon (12 g)	1,344 mcg
Turnip greens	1 cup (180 g)	1,213 mcg
Butter lettuce	1 head	1,123 mcg
Collard greens	1 cup (180 g)	1,106 mcg

BUTYRATE

Why It's Good

Butyrate, also known as butyric acid, is a substance that our colon cells rely on for producing energy. Colon cells will use butyrate preferentially over glutamine and glucose. Through the fermentation process, a certain type of bacteria, called resistant starch, is formed. This type of starch is not digested by the body. Butyrate has several benefits including helping to control blood sugar, reduce constipation, prevent and fight cancer, lower colon inflammation, help break down fat, boost the immune system and prevent heart disease.

Butyrate is only made in our bodies by the fermentation of bacteria from our colon cells. Okay, it sounds a bit gross, but it's the truth. So, the only way for you to naturally consume this essential nutrient is through whole food.

Latest Research on How It Helps Diabetes Prevention

Dietary supplementation of butyrate has been shown to prevent and treat diet-induced insulin resistance. The mechanism of butyrate action is related to the promotion of energy expenditure and induction of mitochondria function.

Best Sources of Butyrate

FOOD	SOURCE OF BUTYRATE
Apples (skin)	Pectin
Whole wheat	Hemicellulose
Barley	Hemicellulose
Rye	Hemicellulose
Oats	Hemicellulose
Bran	Hemicellulose
Mushrooms	Chitin
Legumes (soybeans, lentils, peanuts)	Raffinose, hemicellulose
Fruits and vegetables (found in all whole plant sources, not juice)	Cellulose
Whole grains (bran portion of grain)	Cellulose

OMEGA-3 FATTY ACIDS

Why It's Good

Omega-3 fatty acids are polyunsaturated fatty acids that are essential for optimal health. They are needed in the body to help control blood clotting and build cell membranes in the brain. Omega-3 fatty acids are essential nutrients, which means our bodies are not able to produce them on their own; we must get them from our diet. These fatty acids are also associated with health benefits, including protecting against heart disease, lowering blood triglyceride levels and lowering blood pressure (slightly).

It is always best to increase omega-3 fatty acid consumption through foods first. Try focusing on increasing the variety of omega-3-rich foods in your diet.

People with heart disease may want to talk to their doctor about adding an omega-3 supplement, in addition to their dietary intake of the nutrient. Exceeding recommended intakes of omega-3 supplements can cause excessive bleeding in some people, so make sure to listen to your doctor's recommendations.

Latest Research on How It Helps Diabetes Prevention

Studies have shown that diets rich in omega-3 fatty acids may decrease insulin resistance in people with diabetes. Additionally, people with diabetes often have high triglyceride and low HDL ("good") cholesterol levels. Omega-3 fatty acids from fish oil can help lower triglycerides and raise HDL. Other omega-3 fatty acids (from flaxseeds, etc.) may not have the same benefit as fish oil. According to the American Heart Association, omega-3 fish oil is known to reduce the risk of heart disease as well.

I recommend 3,000 mg of omega-3 fatty acids per day for both men and women.

Best Sources of Omega-3s

FOOD	SERVING	TOTAL OMEGA-3S
Flaxseeds	2 tablespoons (20 g)	3,190 mg
Walnuts	¼ cup (30 g)	2,720 mg
Soybeans	1 cup (200 g)	1,030 mg
Tofu	4 ounces (113 g)	660 mg
Brussels sprouts	1 cup (230 g)	270 mg
Cauliflower	1 cup (230 g)	210 mg
Winter squash	1 cup (200 g)	190 mg
Broccoli	1 cup (230 g)	190 mg
Collard greens	1 cup (180 g)	180 mg
Mustard seeds	2 tablespoons (20 g)	150 mg

Tips: 6 Spices That Help with Blood Sugar Control

Cinnamon: Cinnamon can help to lower blood sugar by decreasing insulin resistance. No study has conclusively proven this; however, it has been noted that most of these studies involved cassia cinnamon (which is also the variety most commonly found at the grocery store), whereas Saigon cinnamon has been observed to be more effective at lowering blood glucose. There are many possible ways to include cinnamon in your diet, such as stirring about half a teaspoon into hot cereal at breakfast or adding it to a banana smoothie. Additionally, cinnamon tea can be purchased, or you can make your own by dropping a cinnamon stick into a cup of unsweetened green or black tea. Cinnamon is also available in supplemental capsules, although these capsules should not be combined with other blood sugar–lowering medications without consulting a doctor first. Individuals with liver defects should not consume large doses of cinnamon.

Turmeric: Turmeric is often used nutritionally for its detoxification and anti-inflammatory properties, and it has been shown to reduce many of the inflammatory reactions that are overactive in diabetes patients. Additionally, it can improve the response of some insulin pathways known to be inhibited in diabetics. Turmeric is most commonly sold as a powder, easily identifiable by its vibrant yellow color, but the root form of this plant can also be found in the produce section of some grocery stores. The powdered spice is mild in flavor and can be mixed into most savory hot foods, especially soups and lentils. One to 3 grams (about 1 teaspoon) per day is recommended.

Ginger: Ginger has been shown to improve insulin sensitivity and has also led to observed improvements in cholesterol and lipid profiles of diabetic patients. Commonly found in grocery stores as both a root and a powdered spice, ginger has many culinary applications. The root is a staple in many juices, used to impart warmth and flavor and to counteract the bitterness of greens. Finely diced ginger root can also be sautéed with garlic and greens, such as kale or bok choy.

Cayenne: Cayenne is a spicy pepper, and studies have shown that capsaicin (the chemical that makes peppers taste spicy) can also help to curb the severity of spikes in blood glucose. Cayenne is most commonly found in its powdered form and can be added to any savory dish to give them more of a kick. Add pinches of cayenne little by little until you reach the desired level of spice.

Parsley: Parsley is an herb that has been shown to decrease blood glucose by enhancing liver function in regard to the interaction between liver cells and insulin. Parsley can be purchased in its dried form but is incredibly easy to find fresh, and there is no upper limit to how much can be consumed each day. Parsley is packed with several nutrients (such as folic acid, vitamins A and C, magnesium and calcium), so it provides benefits beyond blood glucose control. The fresh herb can be used in salads, sandwiches, juices and smoothies to provide nutrition and flavor.

Fennel: Fennel is a root vegetable with a mildly sweet, pleasant licorice-like flavor. It has been shown to help control blood sugar by aiding in the regulation of digestion and gastrointestinal motility. Additionally, fennel itself is a beneficial food to include in a diabetic diet because, like other nonstarchy vegetables, it is low on the glycemic index (GI) and is more conducive to blood glucose control. Fennel is a great way to add some sweetness to foods without adding sugar; it is tasty both raw and cooked. When served raw, fennel is a flavorful addition to salads and juices. An excellent way to cook fennel is to sauté it in a small amount of coconut oil until it softens, then add a drizzle of lemon juice and serve it on its own or as a side dish. Fennel seeds have similar medicinal benefits, though more evidence exists to support a reduction in blood glucose from consuming fennel bulbs.

To-Do List

- ❑ Start adding more leafy greens and teas on a daily basis.
- ❑ Try out a new recipe with one of the recommended spices.
- ❑ Purchase and start taking your supplements.

Daily Supplements

- ❑ Vitamin D: 1,000 IU per day
- ❑ Vitamin B_{12}: 50–100 mcg per day
- ❑ Omega-3 fatty acids: 3,000 mg per day
- ❑ Magnesium: 320–420 mg per day

CHAPTER 5

LIVING
THE BSM LIFE

Do you want to feel better? Do you want to have more energy? Do you want to lose weight? Do you want to lower your blood sugar? Do you want to be off all of your medication?

If you answered yes to any of the above questions, then it is time to get started on the Blood Sugar Miracle way of eating. Think of this as the first step in your journey to better health. It will be a change, and it may take time to get used to, but nothing happens without taking the first step. It is time to start thinking about food in a new way—in terms of being "whole" and "fresh." Open your mind to a whole new world of fruits and vegetables and beans and whole grains. Maybe you start with just trying a new vegetable each week.

HOW TO TRANSITION TO THE BSM WAY

The Blood Sugar Miracle way of eating is a whole foods, plant-based diet for the first 28 days. This way of eating includes lots of fresh vegetables, fruit, beans, nuts, seeds, whole grains and a small amount of healthy fats. After 28 days, you will get the option to add back fish and eggs on an occasional basis. I would like you to stay plant-based; however, I realize that may not be realistic for everyone. The most important things to avoid—and the foods you won't add back in (ever)—are processed foods, sugar-laden sweets and meat.

No matter how big or small, this change will be for you. It is easier to get started if you *have a plan!*

Step 1

Take a look around your pantry and take stock of what is there. Start by throwing away anything that is white and refined and replace the items with whole grains.

WHITE AND REFINED = THROW OUT	NEW GRAINS TO INCLUDE (TO REPLACE THE WHITE ONES)
Crackers made with white or refined flour	Amaranth
White bread, brioche, challah	Barley
White flour	Bulgur
White pasta	Farro
White rice	Millet
White sugar	Quinoa
	Sprouted-grain bread
	Steel-cut oats
	Whole-grain high-fiber crackers

Step 2

Go food shopping for fresh fruits and vegetables and your new grains.

FRUITS TO INCLUDE

- ❑ Apples (small)
- ❑ Berries (all kinds)
- ❑ Clementines
- ❑ Grapefruit (check for interaction with any medication you are on)
- ❑ Kiwis
- ❑ Plums
- ❑ Pomegranates

(continued)

VEGETABLES TO INCLUDE

- ❑ Artichoke
- ❑ Arugula
- ❑ Asparagus
- ❑ Bok choy
- ❑ Broccoli and broccoli sprouts
- ❑ Brussels sprouts
- ❑ Cabbage
- ❑ Carrots
- ❑ Cauliflower
- ❑ Eggplant
- ❑ Endive
- ❑ Kale
- ❑ Leeks
- ❑ Mushrooms
- ❑ Peppers
- ❑ Red onions
- ❑ Romaine lettuce
- ❑ Shallots
- ❑ Spaghetti squash
- ❑ Spinach
- ❑ Water chestnuts

LEGUMES AND OTHER SOURCES OF PROTEIN

- ❑ Black beans
- ❑ Garbanzo beans (chickpeas)
- ❑ Kidney beans
- ❑ Lentils
- ❑ Mung beans
- ❑ Pinto beans
- ❑ Seitan
- ❑ Shirataki noodles
- ❑ Soybeans
- ❑ Tempeh
- ❑ Tofu
- ❑ Veggie burgers

NUTS, SEEDS AND NUT BUTTERS

- ❑ Almond butter
- ❑ Almonds
- ❑ Brazil nuts
- ❑ Chia seeds
- ❑ Flaxseeds
- ❑ Macadamia nuts
- ❑ Peanut butter
- ❑ Pecans
- ❑ Pistachios
- ❑ Pumpkin seeds
- ❑ Sesame seeds (black and white)
- ❑ Soy nut butter
- ❑ Sunflower seeds
- ❑ Walnuts

DAIRY ALTERNATIVES

- ❑ Unsweetened nondairy milks, such as soy, almond or hemp

FATS AND OILS

- ❑ Avocados
- ❑ Fresh olives
- ❑ Oils: avocado, walnut, sesame, flaxseed, extra-virgin olive

Step 3

Start making some of the recipes provided in chapters 7 through 12 of this book.

VISUAL AIDS

Sometimes visual aids can help you identify how much you are eating at a given time. Here are some examples of household items that represent serving sizes of common food items.

FOOD	SIZE
Nonstarchy vegetables	
1 cup (340 g) raw	1 baseball
Grains and starchy vegetables	
½ cup (100 g) beans, peas, lentils	½ baseball
½ cup (80 g) pasta, quinoa, rice	½ baseball
1 slice of bread	1 CD case
Fruit	
1 medium apple, orange, pear	1 baseball
¼ cup (38 g) dried fruit	1 golf ball
Fish	
3 ounces (85 g) (cooked)	1 deck of cards
Dairy alternatives	
1 cup (237 ml) fat-free or low-fat nondairy milk (almond, coconut, etc.)	1 baseball
6 ounces (170 g) low-fat or fat-free nondairy yogurt (almond, coconut, etc.)	1 container
Fats	
¼ cup (30 g) nuts	1 golf ball
1 tablespoon (12 g) peanut or nut butter	½ walnut
1 tablespoon (15 ml) oil	½ shot glass

HOW TO NATURALLY INCREASE THE SWEETNESS OF FOODS

Vanilla powder: Use it as a sweetener. You can buy it in the bean form and crush the beans at home. You can use vanilla or almond extract, but the alcohol in the extract diminishes the sweetness.

All-natural or homemade applesauce: Applesauce can be used as a sugar substitute in baking as it brings a touch of flavor without overwhelming the goods.

Almond milk: Almonds contain minimal sugar, but because of their sweet-tasting oil they can trick our taste buds into thinking sugar is present. Drink it on its own or add it to tea or smoothies. Try to find the unsweetened kind without added sugar—or make it yourself!

Crushed berries: Crush some berries, such as raspberries, blueberries or strawberries, and use it on whole-grain toast or mix into such foods as smoothies. Frozen berries work well as they create their own sauce when thawed. Crushed berries, chopped apple and pear also mix nicely into baked goods.

Avocado: Add avocado to smoothies or use it on salads or in a sandwich. Most store-bought dressings are packed with sugar. Make some at home by mixing mashed avocado, extra-virgin olive oil and some vinegar.

Cinnamon: Add the spice to oatmeal and homemade smoothies for flavor. Try adding a pinch of it to coffee or tea as well.

Coconut flesh and flakes: There is nothing as sweet as raw coconut flesh scooped straight from the coconut, but the other way to eat it is by adding it to cooked oatmeal. If accessing the fresh flesh is not an option, toss in some unsweetened flakes.

Cooked onion: Many savory foods, such as pasta sauce and soup, have added sugar. This is especially true for foods with a tomato base, due to tomatoes' acidity. Use onion instead of sugar; let the onions caramelize by sautéing on the stovetop until they're deeply golden.

Roasted vegetables: Roasting vegetables with a bit of extra-virgin olive oil and salt can make them extremely sweet. The most dessertlike vegetables are sweet potato, squash, beets and carrots. Eat the roasted vegetables at the end of the meal, and you will be far less tempted to need something sweet.

Prunes or dates: Get out your blender and puree prunes and dates to add natural sweetness and nutritional power to baked goods, also allowing you to omit sugar in the recipe.

Tips to Get Started

1. Don't think of it as a big change. Think about the meals you already eat that are meatless, such as eggplant Parmesan, rice and beans, and pasta with marinara sauce.

2. Try out some new recipes.

3. You can make almost any meal that you already eat and just take out the meat. For example, you can make vegetarian fajitas instead of beef fajitas or a three-bean chili instead of a meat chili.

4. To save time, make up larger batches of foods—for example, lentils or vegetable soups or veggie burgers—and freeze them. Then you can just heat and eat.

5. Try one new vegetable or recipe per week.

DINING OUT GUIDE

You can still eat out and enjoy the benefits of restaurant dining and follow the BSM way. Let the following suggestions for dining out help you make smart food choices.

Regardless of the cuisine, there are always healthy (or healthier) options on any restaurant menu. In addition to the food choice, consider the following tips:

1. Ask for half-portions of a food item, or ask the portion to be split before serving so you can easily take the second half home.
2. Consider ordering an appetizer as your main course. These are often much smaller portions than the main courses, less expensive and just as tasty!
3. Drink a glass of water right when you sit down at the table.

American

AVOID	CHOOSE
Items with the words fried, crispy, deep-fried, battered, jumbo or stacked in the title	Green salad. Ask for oil and vinegar or a low-calorie vinaigrette on the side and no cheese.
Creamy dressings or cream-based soups	Veggie burger loaded with greens. Replace French fries or chips with a side salad or vegetable.
	Vegetable, lentil or bean soup
	Roasted, baked or steamed fish with steamed vegetables and quinoa (after the first 28 days)

Italian

AVOID	CHOOSE
Breadbaskets before the meal or garlic bread	Side salad to start, with low-calorie vinaigrette or oil and vinegar on the side
Cream or cheese sauces, such as Alfredo	Baked or broiled fish with beans and vegetables (after 28 days)
Sausage, prosciutto or breaded meats	Vegetarian pasta dishes (whole wheat pasta is best) with tomato-based sauces, such as marinara and pomodoro (e.g., pasta primavera)
Anything carbonara or parmigiana	

Mexican

AVOID	CHOOSE
Chips and salsa to start	Appetizers such as black bean soup or gazpacho
Refried beans, pinto beans, cheese and sour cream as toppings	Fish or vegetable tacos or fajitas with corn tortillas (after 28 days)
Excessive portions of guacamole	Toppings such as salad greens, black beans and/or pico de gallo
Fried dishes, such as chiles rellenos, chimachangas or flautas, or hard-shell tacos	Guacamole in moderation
Oversized entrées, such as burritos	Ceviche (after 28 days)

Chinese

AVOID	CHOOSE
Options with fried noodles, fried rice or deep-fried meats	Dishes with vegetables and tofu or fish (after 28 days)
Egg foo yong	Steamed or broiled items
Sweet-and-sour or lobster sauce	Sauces on the side
Deep-fried appetizers, such as egg rolls, scallion pancakes or crab rangoon	Stir-fried vegetable dishes

Indian or Middle Eastern

AVOID	CHOOSE
Food cooked in coconut oil or cream, or containing ghee (clarified butter)	Tandoori vegetables, chana masala, mattar tofu
Tahini/sesame pastes, samosas, pakoras, poori, paratha or phyllo dough	Either basmati or brown rice
Panfried dishes	Fava beans, mashed garbanzo beans (chickpeas) or smoked eggplant

Thai

AVOID	CHOOSE
Coconut-based soups and curries	Hot and sour (tom yum) soup
Peanut sauces	Steamed fish or rice (after 28 days)
	Stir-fried vegetables or fish (after 28 days)

Japanese

AVOID	CHOOSE
Sushi or sashimi with spicy or tempura in the title, or that contain cream cheese or mayonnaise	Miso soup, green or hijiki salads or edamame to start
Excessive use of soy sauce	Sushi or sashimi flavored with ginger and wasabi
Fried dishes, such as agemono, katsu, or tempura	Brown rice as a substitute for white rice in sushi rolls
	Low-sodium soy sauce (still limit this)

How to Handle Travel

- ❏ Always travel with snacks, such as packs of nuts, homemade energy bars and apples.
- ❏ In the airport, look for salad bars, soup or stir-fry restaurants.
- ❏ If traveling internationally, request a vegetarian meal.
- ❏ Bring your own meals as much as possible.

How to Handle a Wedding Reception or Cocktail Party

- ❏ Stock up on such appetizers as crudités, sushi/sashimi or a small dish of pasta. You may have to make the appetizers your main meal.
- ❏ Start with soup or salad.
- ❏ Dance when they serve cake.
- ❏ Sip champagne for the toast.

How to Handle Dinner at a Friend's House

- ❏ Offer to bring a dish (at least you know you will be able to eat something).
- ❏ Load up on veggies and salad.
- ❏ Have fruit for dessert.

THE IMPORTANCE OF WATER

Drinking enough water is essential to our health. The human body is composed of about 60 percent water and depends on water to function at its best.

Water is responsible for flushing toxins from our bodies, carrying nutrients to our cells, lubricating joints, helping to convert food into energy, regulating body temperature and helping to decrease premenstrual bloating.

You should drink at least eight 8-ounce (227-ml) glasses of water every day! This may increase, depending on your physical activity level, the climate you live in, your health status and whether you are pregnant or breastfeeding.

Tips

1. It is important to replace water losses to stay properly hydrated.
2. It can be easy to mistake thirst for hunger, which means you may eat when you are really just dehydrated and thirsty.
3. Choose water first!
4. Try adding a splash of citrus to water or tea for added flavor with no added calories.

To-Do List

- ❏ Clean out your pantry—remove all white and overly processed foods.
- ❏ Go food shopping for your new food groups.
- ❏ Drink 64 ounces of water per day.
- ❏ Keep a list of all the recipes that you have tried and liked that don't contain meat.
- ❏ By the end of the week, you should be having almost all meatless meals.

CHAPTER 6

THE BSM EATING GUIDE

Eating the BSM way will take some cooking and planning. There is no way around it. But you will feel much better and be much happier with yourself, your weight and your blood sugar once you start to get into this way of eating. It is easy to follow the meal plan as all of the recipes are in the book, and there is a week-by-week shopping list.

I realize life could get in the way, and you may not be able to make all of your meals every week. Which is why it is important to understand how many carbohydrates your body needs (Chapter 2) and to understand the foods to choose and foods to avoid, so that if you aren't able to cook everything for that week, you will still be able to follow the BSM plan and get the same great results.

Another option is to use the following tables but mix and match and create your own meal plan for more flexibility. In addition, there are suggestions for meals on the go.

THE BSM 28-DAY PLAN

Phase 1: Foods to Include/Avoid for the First 28 Days

FOODS TO EAT	
Meat substitutes	Seitan, Tempeh, Tofu. Vegan protein power (e.g., Vega One)
Vegetables and legumes	Alfalfa sprouts, arugula, asparagus, bamboo shoots, bell peppers (any color), broccoli, Brussels sprouts, cabbage, carrots, cauliflower, Chinese cabbage, chives, collard greens, cucumbers, eggplant, endive, escarole, garlic, green beans, kale, loose-leaf lettuce (red or green), mustard greens, jicama, mung bean sprouts, mushrooms, okra, onions, parsley, radicchio, radishes, romaine lettuce, spinach, Swiss chard, tomatoes, water chestnuts, watercress, yellow squash, zucchini
Fruits	All fruits (except banana, grapes, mangoes)
Beans	Black-eyed peas, French beans, garbanzo beans (chickpeas) kidney beans, lentils, pinto beans, soybeans, white beans
Whole grains	Amaranth, barley, brown rice, buckwheat, bulgur, millet, oats, quinoa, sweet potato, whole wheat pasta, wild rice
Fats	Oils: coconut, flaxseed, extra-virgin olive. Nuts: almonds, Brazil nuts, macadamia nuts, peanuts (really a legume), pine nuts, pistachios, walnuts. Seeds: chia seeds, flaxseeds, pumpkin seeds, sesame seeds. Nut butter: natural almond or peanut butter. Approved salad dressings
Herbs, spices and seasonings	All spices that contain no added sugar: anise, basil, bay leaves, black pepper, cayenne pepper, chile peppers, cider vinegar, cilantro, cinnamon, cloves, coriander, cumin, dried mustard, dill, fennel, garlic, ginger, parsley, salt, turmeric
Condiments	Horseradish, mustard, pico de gallo, salsa
Extracts	Almond or vanilla

FOODS TO AVOID	
Beef	All types, including brisket, hamburgers, liver, sirloin, steaks, tenderloin, top round
Poultry	All types of poultry, including chicken, duck, goose, turkey bacon, turkey and chicken breast
Eggs	All types
Seafood	All types of fish and shellfish
Pork	All types
Veal	All types
Cheese	All types
Starches	White bread, processed breakfast cereals, white rice, white pasta, and all baked goods, snack foods
Dairy	All dairy, including ice cream, milk and yogurt (does not include soy, almond or coconut milk, yogurt or cheese), powdered milk substitutes and coffee sweeteners, half-and-half
Fruits	All fruit juice. Bananas, grapes, mangoes
Sweets and sweeteners	Sugar, powdered sweetener, artificial sweetener (except stevia). Candies, including sugar-free candy. Commercially prepared cakes, cookies, pies, tarts. Foods containing artificial sweeteners (Splenda, saccharin, Equal, Sweet'N Low, aspartame). Foods containing sugar alcohols: (names that end in -ol or -ose), dextrose, glucose, mannitol, mannose, sorbitol, sucralose, xylitol, xylose. Corn syrup, high-fructose corn syrup, maltodextrin

AVOID THESE INGREDIENTS

- ❏ Alanine/amino acids
- ❏ Albumen
- ❏ Artificial color, FD&C color
- ❏ Aspartic acid
- ❏ BHA
- ❏ BHT
- ❏ Casein
- ❏ Fatty acids
- ❏ Gelatin, gel
- ❏ Glycerin, glycerol
- ❏ Lactic acid
- ❏ Lactose
- ❏ Lard
- ❏ Lecithin
- ❏ Lipase
- ❏ Lipoids
- ❏ Methionine
- ❏ Monoglycerides
- ❏ MSG
- ❏ Nitrates
- ❏ Oleic acid
- ❏ Olestra
- ❏ Polysorbates
- ❏ Potassium bromate
- ❏ Rapeseed oil
- ❏ Rennet
- ❏ Saccharine
- ❏ Stearic acid
- ❏ Tallow, fatty alcohol
- ❏ Urea, uric acid
- ❏ Whey

Phase 2: Foods to Include/Avoid after the First 28 Days

All the same ones as in Phase 1.

Reintroduce fish/seafood, egg whites and Greek yogurt on an occasional basis.

THE BSM 28-DAY MENU

Start off each day with 8 ounces of Daily Detox Elixir (page 160). Add 1 teaspoon (5 g) of flaxseed oil or 4 teaspoons (20 g) of ground flaxseeds to any meal or beverage throughout the day. Keep reading for your shopping list (page 74) and the recipes (starting on page 82). When more than one snack is listed, please enjoy both.

Week 1

	BREAKFAST	LUNCH	SNACK	DINNER
DAY 1	Lemon Avocado Toast (page 84)	Curly Kale Salad (page 99)	**Snack 1:** 1 green apple with 20 almonds **Snack 2:** ¾ cup (114 g) strawberries	Ginger-Lemongrass Stir-fry (page 129) over ½ cup (80 g) cooked quinoa
Daily Nutrient Analysis: Calories: 1303, Fat: 72.6 g, Carbohydrates: 139.1 g, Fiber: 35.7 g, Net Carbohydrates: 103.4 g, Protein: 36.6 g				
DAY 2	Berry Bliss Smoothie (page 87)	Cali Bean Burger (page 111) on a 6″ (15 cm) sprouted-wheat tortilla; Summer Gazpacho (page 115)	Apple Cinnamon Bars (page 146) with ¾ cup (102 g) blueberries	Zucchini Spaghetti with Vegetable Marinara (page 117); Harissa-Spiced White Bean and Vegetable "Mash" (page 127)
Daily Nutrient Analysis: Calories: 1243, Fat: 46.1 g, Carbohydrates: 150.3 g, Fiber: 36.3 g, Net Carbohydrates: 116 g, Protein: 68.8 g				
DAY 3	Perfect Almond Berry Parfait (page 86)	Avocado and Tomato Sandwich (page 106); Glowing Green Seaweed Salad (page 149)	Rainbow Chard Chips (page 138) with 1 pear	Miso-Marinated Tofu with Sesame Broccoli (page 125) over ½ cup (80 g) cooked quinoa
Daily Nutrient Analysis: Calories: 1229, Fat: 56.2 g, Carbohydrates: 139.2 g, Fiber: 38.7 g, Net Carbohydrates: 10.5 g, Protein: 48.6 g				
DAY 4	Energizing Açai Bowl (page 85)	Arugula and Wild Mushroom Salad with Citrus-Walnut Dressing (page 98); top with 4 ounces (113 g) tofu	**Snack 1:** 45 pistachios with 1 green apple **Snack 2:** 3 Peanut Butter Bites (page 144)	Skinny Eggplant Parmesan (page 121) with Sautéed Tuscan Kale (page 152)
Daily Nutrient Analysis: Calories: 1359, Fat: 71.7 g, Carbohydrates: 145.7 g, Fiber: 36.1 g, Net Carbohydrates: 111.6 g, Protein: 50 g				
DAY 5	Green Goddess Smoothie (page 88)	Southwestern Salad (page 97)	**Snack 1:** Green Vitality Toast with Chili-Lime Salt (page 140) **Snack 2:** 20 almonds	Cauliflower and Leek Soup (page 110) with Quinoa-Stuffed Bell Peppers (page 123)
Daily Nutrient Analysis: Calories: 1357, Fat: 55.7 g, Carbohydrates: 165 g, Fiber: 39 g, Net Carbohydrates: 98.9 g, Protein: 49.2 g				
DAY 6	Sunny Scrambled Tofu with Market Vegetables (page 91) and 1 slice whole-grain toast	Autumn Harvest Chickpea Salad (page 101); 1 cup (136 g) Chickpea Soup (page 108)	**Snack 1:** Chia Seed Pudding (page 94) **Snack 2:** 1 green apple	Vegetable Lasagne with Cashew Ricotta (page 122); Glowing Green Seaweed Salad (page 149)
Daily Nutrient Analysis: Calories: 1483, Fat: 70.6 g, Carbohydrates: 153.5 g, Fiber: 42.9 g, Net Carbohydrates: 110.6 g, Protein: 63.8 g				
DAY 7	Strawberry–Almond Butter Pancakes (page 83)	Portobello Kimchi Lettuce Wraps (page 105)	1 green apple with 20 almonds	Outrageously Good Homemade Veggie Burgers (page 119); Cooling Cucumber Salad (page 150)
Daily Nutrient Analysis: Calories: 1368, Fat: 75.8 g, Carbohydrates: 136.5 g, Fiber: 40.8 g, Net Carbohydrates: 95.7 g, Protein: 53.1 g				

Week 2

	BREAKFAST	LUNCH	SNACK	DINNER
DAY 8	Morning Warrior Bars (page 93) with 1 green apple	Eat out (Japanese): miso soup, green salad with ginger dressing; brown rice and avocado roll; shiitake mushroom and cucumber roll (no rice, wrapped in cucumber)	45 pistachios with 1 pear	One-Pot Vegetarian Sauté (page 128)

Daily Nutrient Analysis: Calories: 1513, Fat: 54.1 g, Carbohydrates: 211.7 g, Fiber: 33 g, Net Carbohydrates: 178.7 g, Protein: 47.6 g

	BREAKFAST	LUNCH	SNACK	DINNER
DAY 9	Extremely Tasty Vegetable "Frittata" (page 92)	Dinosaur Kale Salad with Asian Pear and Pomegranate Vinaigrette (page 114) and 4 ounces (113 g) tofu	**Snack 1:** 1 cup (136 g) edamame (in the shell) with ¾ cup (102 g) blueberries

Snack 2: 1 Apple Cinnamon Bars (page 146) | Spicy Chana Masala (page 120) |

Daily Nutrient Analysis: Calories. 1265, Fat: 59.1 g, Carbohydrates: 136.4 g, Fiber: 34.8 g, Net Carbohydrates: 101.6 g, Protein: 59.7 g

	BREAKFAST	LUNCH	SNACK	DINNER
DAY 10	Green Goddess Smoothie (page 88)	Winter White Bean Soup with Kale and Basil Pistou (page 103); Cali Bean Burger (page 111) on a 6" (15 cm) sprouted-wheat tortilla	Rainbow Chard Chips (page 138)	Black Bean and Roasted Vegetable Quesadilla with Spicy Pico de Gallo (page 126)

Daily Nutrient Analysis: Calories: 1097, Fat: 51.2 g, Carbohydrates: 1543 g, Fiber: 33 g, Net Carbohydrates: 111 g, Protein: 41.2 g

	BREAKFAST	LUNCH	SNACK	DINNER
DAY 11	Energizing Açai Bowl (page 85)	Zesty Tomato and Avocado Tartine (page 100); Cauliflower and Leek Soup (page 110)	**Snack 1:** Crunchy Chickpeas (page 147)

Snack 2: 2 clementines with 20 almonds | Vegetable Lasagne with Cashew Ricotta (page 122) |

Daily Nutrient Analysis: Calories: 1499, Fat: 58.9 g, Carbohydrates: 199.7 g, Fiber: 48.3 g, Net Carbohydrates: 151.4 g, Protein: 53.8 g

	BREAKFAST	LUNCH	SNACK	DINNER
DAY 12	Spiced Steel-Cut Oats (page 90)	Curried Tofu Pita Pockets (page 104); Glowing Green Seaweed Salad (page 149)	**Snack 1:** almond milk yogurt with ½ cup (68 g) blueberries

Snack 2: 3 Peanut Butter Bites (page 144) | Roasted Portobello Burger (page 124); Lemony Brussels Sprouts (page 151) |

Daily Nutrient Analysis: Calories: 1401, Fat: 71.9 g, Carbohydrates: 156.5 g, Fiber: 55 g, Net Carbohydrates: 101.5, Protein: 61 g

	BREAKFAST	LUNCH	SNACK	DINNER
DAY 13	2 slices multigrain toast, 2 tablespoons (30 g) Cashew Dream Cheese (page 171) topped with 4 slices each tomato and red onion	Mini Baked Falafel Burgers in Lettuce Cups with Cucumber-Yogurt Sauce (page 102)	**Snack 1:** 1 Vegan Pumpkin Muffins (page 95) with 1 green apple

Snack 2: 1 green apple with 20 almonds | Miso-Marinated Tofu with Sesame Broccoli (page 125); Spicy Ginger Baby Bok Choy (page 155); ½ cup (80 g) cooked quinoa |

Daily Nutrient Analysis: Calories: 1233, Fat: 55 g, Carbohydrates: 148.6 g, Fiber: 31.3 g, Net Carbohydrates: 117.3 g, Protein: 49.5 g

	BREAKFAST	LUNCH	SNACK	DINNER
DAY 14	Strawberry–Almond Butter Pancakes (page 83)	Guiltless Seitan "BLT" Pockets (page 109)	Nirvana Chips (page 139)	Louisiana Red Beans and Smoked Tempeh with Quinoa and Swiss Chard Sauté (page 118)

Daily Nutrient Analysis: Calories: 1567, Fat: 83.8 g, Carbohydrates: 103.5 g, Fiber: 22.8 g, Net Carbohydrates: 94.7 g, Protein: 97.1 g

Week 3

	BREAKFAST	LUNCH	SNACK	DINNER
DAY 15	2 slices whole-grain bread topped with 1 tablespoon (9 g) almond butter and ½ cup (68 g) blueberries	Southwestern Salad (page 97)	1 green apple with Spicy Popcorn (page 137)	Ginger-Lemongrass Stir-fry (page 129) and ½ cup (80 g) cooked quinoa
Daily Nutrient Analysis: Calories: 1394, Fat: 62 g, Carbohydrates: 178.2 g, Fiber: 54.6, Net Carbohydrates: 141.6, Protein: 40.7 g				
DAY 16	Lemon Avocado Toast (page 84)	Curried Tofu Pita Pockets (page 104)	1 cup (136 g) carrots with 2 tablespoons (17 g) Za'atar-Flaxseed Hummus (page 131)	Zucchini Spaghetti with Vegetable Marinara (page 117); Harissa-Spiced White Bean and Vegetable "Mash" (page 127)
Daily Nutrient Analysis: Calories: 1393, Fat: 62.8 g, Carbohydrates: 140.4 g, Fiber: 41.2 g, Net Carbohydrates: 99.2 g, Protein: 77.6 g				
DAY 17	Vegan Pumpkin Muffins (page 95) with 1 green apple	Portobello Kimchi Lettuce Wraps (page 105); Cooling Cucumber Salad (page 150)	2 Antioxidant Chocolate Coins (page 145) and 1 cup (151 g) of strawberries	Outrageously Good Homemade Veggie Burgers (page 119); Sautéed Tuscan Kale (page 152); Creamy Cauliflower Mashed Potatoes (page 158)
Daily Nutrient Analysis: Calories: 1298, Fat: 63.7 g, Carbohydrates: 158.5 g, Fiber: 42.5 g, Net Carbohydrates: 116 g, Protein: 42.6 g				
DAY 18	Spiced Steel-Cut Oats (page 90) with toasted almonds	Dinosaur Kale Salad with Asian Pear and Pomegranate Vinaigrette (page 114)	**Snack 1:** 1 cup (136 g) Crunchy Chickpeas (page 147) **Snack 2:** 1 Apple Cinnamon Bars (page 146)	Vegetable Lasagne with Cashew Ricotta (page 122); Cooling Cucumber Salad (page 150)
Daily Nutrient Analysis: Calories: 1230, Fat: 61.5 g, Carbohydrates: 145.9 g, Fiber: 29.5 g, Net Carbohydrates: 116.4 g, Protein: 40.2 g				
DAY 19	Berry Bliss Smoothie (page 87)	Chickpea Soup (page 108) with a green salad and Citrus Walnut Dressing (page 98)	3 pieces of bran crispbread spread with 2 tablespoons (17 g) Eggplant Spread (page 132)	Black Bean and Roasted Vegetable Quesadilla with Spicy Pico de Gallo (page 126); Glowing Green Seaweed Salad (page 149)
Daily Nutrient Analysis: Calories: 1457, Fat: 85.4 g, Carbohydrates: 153.4 g, Fiber: 59.5 g, Net Carbohydrates: 94 g, Protein: 47.3 g				
DAY 20	Extremely Tasty Vegetable "Frittata" (page 92)	Avocado and Tomato Sandwich (page 106); Summer Gazpacho (page 115)	Green Goddess Smoothie (page 88)	Louisiana Red Beans and Smoked Tempeh with Quinoa and Swiss Chard Sauté (page 118)
Daily Nutrient Analysis: Calories: 1618, Fat: 68.4 g, Carbohydrates: 156.5 g, Fiber: 39.6 g, Net Carbohydrates: 130.9 g, Protein: 77.2 g				
DAY 21	Chia Seed Pudding (page 94) with 1 cup (151 g) strawberries	Winter White Bean Soup with Kale and Basil Pistou (page 103); Cali Bean Burger (without bread) (page 111)	Strawberry Smoothie (page 143)	Eating Out (Chinese): broccoli with tofu in garlic sauce over 1 cup (160 g) brown rice
Daily Nutrient Analysis: Calories: 1411, Fat: 67.3 g, Carbohydrates: 170.6 g, Fiber: 34.2 g, Net Carbohydrates: 143.4 g, Protein: 44.6 g				

Week 4

WEEK 4	BREAKFAST	LUNCH	SNACK	DINNER
DAY 22	Energizing Açai Bowl (page 85)	Spicy Tempeh Salad (page 113)	1 green apple with 1 tablespoon (15 g) almond butter	Outrageously Good Homemade Veggie Burgers (page 119); Cooling Cucumber Salad (page 150)
Daily Nutrient Analysis: Calories: 1377, Fat: 73.6 g, Carbohydrates: 136.5 g, Fiber: 38.7 g, Net Carbohydrates: 104.8 g, Protein: 47.6 g				
DAY 23	Perfect Almond Berry Parfait (page 86)	Vegetarian Quinoa and Black Bean Wraps (page 107); Chickpea Soup (page 108)	**Snack 1:** 3 pieces of bran crispbread with ⅓ avocado (mashed) and 3 slices of tomato **Snack 2:** 1 cup (151 g) strawberries with 20 almonds	Skinny Eggplant Parmesan (page 121); Sautéed Tuscan Kale (page 152)
Daily Nutrient Analysis: Calories: 1296, Fat: 59.2 g, Carbohydrates: 159.8 g, Fiber: 39.7 g, Net Carbohydrates: 122.1 g, Protein: 52.2 g				
DAY 24	Morning Warrior Bars (page 93) with 1 green apple	Autumn Harvest Chickpea Salad (page 101) with 4 ounces (113 g) tofu	½ cup (68 g) Granola Clusters (page 142) with ½ cup (68 g) blueberries	Vegetable Lasagne with Cashew Ricotta (page 122)
Daily Nutrient Analysis: Calories: 1279, Fat: 67.7 g, Carbohydrates: 133.7 g, Fiber: 26.6 g, Net Carbohydrates: 107.1 g, Protein: 53.1 g				
DAY 25	Green Goddess Smoothie (page 88)	Baked Falafel Burgers in Lettuce Cups with Yogurt Cucumber Yogurt Sauce (page 102)	45 pistachios; 1 green apple	One-Pot Vegetarian Sauté (page 128); Arugula and Wild Mushroom Salad with Citrus-Walnut Dressing (page 98)
Daily Nutrient Analysis: Calories: 1133, Fat: 37.7 g, Carbohydrates: 144 g, Fiber: 28 g, Net Carbohydrates: 116 g, Protein: 50.2 g				
DAY 26	Chia Seed Pudding (page 94) with 1 cup (157 g) strawberries	Zesty Tomato and Avocado Tartine (page 100) with Cauliflower and Leek Soup (page 110)	**Snack 1:** 3 Peanut Butter Bites (page 144) with 2 clementines **Snack 2:** Apple Cinnamon Bars (page 146)	Quinoa-Stuffed Bell Peppers (page 123) with Glowing Green Seaweed Salad (page 149)
Daily Nutrient Analysis: Calories: 1391, Fat: 62.1 g, Carbohydrates: 176.1 g, Fiber: 41 g, Net Carbohydrates: 135.1 g, Protein: 43.1 g				
DAY 27	Berry Bliss Smoothie (page 87)	Guiltless Seitan "BLT" Pockets (page 109)	**Snack 1:** 1 Vegan Pumpkin Muffins (page 95) with ½ cup (68 g) blueberries **Snack 2:** 1 pear	Ginger-Lemongrass Stir-fry (page 129) with ¼ cup (50 g) cubed baked tofu and ½ cup (80 g) cooked quinoa
Daily Nutrient Analysis: Calories: 1212, Fat: 45.9 g, Carbohydrates: 139.2 g, Fiber: 25.7 g, Net Carbohydrates: 113.5 g, Protein: 72.4 g				
DAY 28	Sunny Scrambled Tofu with Market Vegetables (page 91)	Curried Tofu Pita Pockets (page 104)	**Snack 1:** 3 pieces bran crispbread with 2 tablespoons (17 g) Eggplant Spread (page 132) **Snack 2:** 45 pistachios	Black Bean and Roasted Vegetable Quesadilla with Spicy Pico de Gallo (page 126)
Daily Nutrient Analysis: Calories: 1167, Fat: 70.8 g, Carbohydrates: 116.5 g, Fiber: 42.7 g, Net Carbohydrates: 74.8 g, Protein: 65.5 g				

Following are week-by-week shopping lists for all the necessary ingredients to prepare a month's worth of menus. See the appendix for some recommended brands of store-bought products, such as breads.

28-DAY MEAL PLAN SHOPPING LIST (WEEKLY)

Shopping List for Phase 1 Meal Plan

Everyday Staples to Always Have on Hand

HERBS & SPICES

- ❑ Black pepper
- ❑ Cajun seasoning
- ❑ Cayenne pepper
- ❑ Chili powder
- ❑ Crushed red pepper flakes
- ❑ Curry powder
- ❑ Dried oregano
- ❑ Dried parsley
- ❑ Dried rosemary
- ❑ Dried sage
- ❑ Dried thyme
- ❑ Fennel seeds
- ❑ Garlic powder
- ❑ Ground cinnamon
- ❑ Ground cloves
- ❑ Ground coriander
- ❑ Ground cumin
- ❑ Ground ginger
- ❑ Ground nutmeg
- ❑ Herbes de Provence
- ❑ Old Bay seasoning
- ❑ Onion powder
- ❑ Paprika
- ❑ Pumpkin pie spice
- ❑ Salt
- ❑ Sesame seeds (white, black)
- ❑ Turmeric

OILS

- ❑ Coconut oil
- ❑ Extra-virgin olive oil
- ❑ Hazelnut oil
- ❑ Sesame oil
- ❑ Walnut oil

SWEETENERS/BAKING NEEDS

- ❑ Agave nectar
- ❑ All-purpose flour
- ❑ Baking powder
- ❑ Baking soda
- ❑ Cornstarch
- ❑ Golden brown sugar
- ❑ Honey
- ❑ Nutritional yeast
- ❑ Vanilla extract

VINEGARS

- ❑ Balsamic vinegar
- ❑ Cider vinegar
- ❑ Red wine vinegar
- ❑ Rice vinegar
- ❑ Sherry vinegar

CONDIMENTS

- ❑ Dijon mustard
- ❑ Hot sauce
- ❑ Mirin
- ❑ Tahini
- ❑ White miso
- ❑ Whole-grain mustard
- ❑ Wine (dry white, red)
- ❑ Worcestershire sauce

Week 1 Shopping List

PRODUCE

- ❑ Apples (green, Fuji)
- ❑ Arugula
- ❑ Avocados
- ❑ Bananas
- ❑ Bell peppers (red, yellow)
- ❑ Blueberries
- ❑ Broccoli
- ❑ Butter lettuce
- ❑ Carrots
- ❑ Cauliflower
- ❑ Celery
- ❑ Chinese broccoli
- ❑ Cucumber (English, Japanese)
- ❑ Eggplant
- ❑ Garlic
- ❑ Ginger
- ❑ Jalapeño chiles
- ❑ Kale (curly, Tuscan, dinosaur, baby)
- ❑ Kiwis
- ❑ Leeks
- ❑ Lemons
- ❑ Limes
- ❑ Mushrooms (cremini, shiitake, portobello)
- ❑ Onions (red, yellow)
- ❑ Oranges
- ❑ Pears
- ❑ Rainbow chard
- ❑ Raspberries
- ❑ Roasted red peppers
- ❑ Romaine lettuce
- ❑ Scallions
- ❑ Shallots
- ❑ Snow peas
- ❑ Spinach
- ❑ Strawberries
- ❑ Sun-dried tomatoes
- ❑ Tomatoes (Roma, heirloom, cherry)
- ❑ Zucchini

FRESH HERBS

- ❑ Cilantro
- ❑ Dill
- ❑ Lemongrass
- ❑ Parsley
- ❑ Rosemary
- ❑ Shiso
- ❑ Thyme

GRAINS

- ❑ Healthy Joy Omega Power Bread
- ❑ Quinoa
- ❑ Rolled oats
- ❑ Sprouted-grain bread
- ❑ Sprouted-grain tortillas
- ❑ Steel-cut oats

DAIRY ALTERNATIVES

- ❑ Almond milk, unsweetened
- ❑ Almond milk yogurt, plain
- ❑ Soy milk, unsweetened

PROTEINS

- ❑ Almond butter
- ❑ Almond slivers
- ❑ Lentils
- ❑ Low-sodium black beans
- ❑ Low-sodium cannellini beans
- ❑ Low-sodium garbanzo beans (chickpeas)
- ❑ Low-sodium pinto beans
- ❑ Low-sodium red kidney beans
- ❑ Raw almonds
- ❑ Raw cashews
- ❑ Seitan
- ❑ Tempeh
- ❑ Tofu (extra-firm, silken)
- ❑ Unsalted pistachios
- ❑ Unsalted, creamy peanut butter (all-natural)

(continued)

- ❑ Açai, frozen
- ❑ Almond flour
- ❑ Almond meal
- ❑ Bamboo shoots
- ❑ Capers
- ❑ Chipotle chiles in adobe sauce
- ❑ Dried figs
- ❑ Dried seaweed
- ❑ Flaxseeds
- ❑ Harissa
- ❑ Homemade granola
- ❑ Low-sodium V8 juice
- ❑ Matcha powder
- ❑ Panko bread crumbs
- ❑ San Marzano tomatoes
- ❑ Unsweetened coconut flakes
- ❑ Vegan mayonnaise
- ❑ Vegetable stock
- ❑ Whole wheat bread crumbs

Week 2 Shopping List

PRODUCE

- ❑ Apples (green, Gala)
- ❑ Arugula
- ❑ Asparagus
- ❑ Avocados
- ❑ Baby bok choy
- ❑ Banana
- ❑ Bell peppers (red, green)
- ❑ Blueberries
- ❑ Carrots
- ❑ Cauliflower
- ❑ Celery
- ❑ Chinese broccoli
- ❑ Cilantro
- ❑ Clementines
- ❑ Cucumbers
- ❑ Dates
- ❑ Fennel
- ❑ Garlic
- ❑ Ginger
- ❑ Jalapeño chiles
- ❑ Kale (dinosaur, red Russian, Tuscan, baby)
- ❑ Kiwis
- ❑ Leeks
- ❑ Lemons
- ❑ Limes
- ❑ Mushrooms (cremini, portobello)
- ❑ Onions (red, yellow)
- ❑ Pomegranate arils
- ❑ Rainbow chard
- ❑ Romaine
- ❑ Scallions
- ❑ Serrano chile
- ❑ Spinach
- ❑ Strawberries
- ❑ Sweet potatoes
- ❑ Tomatoes
- ❑ Zucchini

FRESH HERBS

- ❑ Basil
- ❑ Parsley
- ❑ Rosemary
- ❑ Thyme

GRAINS

- ❑ Low-carb pita pockets
- ❑ Quinoa
- ❑ Rolled oats

- ❑ Sprouted-grain bread and tortilla
- ❑ Sprouted-grain tortillas
- ❑ Steel-cut oats

DAIRY ALTERNATIVES

- ❑ Almond milk, unsweetened
- ❑ Almond milk yogurt, plain
- ❑ Hazelnut milk, unsweetened

PROTEINS

- ❑ Almond slivers
- ❑ Dry-roasted peanuts, unsalted
- ❑ Green lentils
- ❑ Low-sodium black beans
- ❑ Low-sodium cannellini beans
- ❑ Low sodium garbanzo beans (chickpeas)
- ❑ Low-sodium red kidney beans
- ❑ Peanut butter (all-natural)
- ❑ Raw almonds
- ❑ Raw cashews
- ❑ Seitan
- ❑ Tempeh
- ❑ Tofu (extra-firm, silken)
- ❑ Unsalted pistachios

GROCERY

- ❑ Açai, frozen
- ❑ Almond flour
- ❑ Almond meal
- ❑ Chipotle chiles in adobe sauce
- ❑ Dried figs
- ❑ Dried seaweed
- ❑ Edamame
- ❑ Flaxseeds
- ❑ Garbanzo bean flour
- ❑ Kalamata olives
- ❑ Peaches, frozen
- ❑ Protein powder
- ❑ Pumpkin puree
- ❑ Pumpkin seeds
- ❑ Roasted red peppers
- ❑ San Marzano tomatoes
- ❑ Unsweetened coconut flakes
- ❑ Vegan mayonnaise
- ❑ Vegetable stock
- ❑ Wasabi powder

Week 3 Shopping List

PRODUCE

- ❑ Apples (green, Gala)
- ❑ Asian pears
- ❑ Asparagus
- ❑ Avocados
- ❑ Bananas
- ❑ Bell peppers (red, green)
- ❑ Blueberries
- ❑ Carrots
- ❑ Cauliflower
- ❑ Celery
- ❑ Cucumber (English, Japanese)
- ❑ Dates
- ❑ Eggplant
- ❑ Garlic
- ❑ Ginger
- ❑ Jalapeño chiles
- ❑ Kale (baby, Tuscan, dinosaur, Red Russian)
- ❑ Lemons
- ❑ Limes
- ❑ Mushrooms (cremini, shiitake, portobello)
- ❑ Onions (red, yellow)
- ❑ Pears
- ❑ Pomegranate arils
- ❑ Raspberries
- ❑ Romaine lettuce

(continued)

- ❑ Scallion
- ❑ Serrano chiles
- ❑ Shallots
- ❑ Snow peas
- ❑ Spinach
- ❑ Strawberries
- ❑ Swiss chard
- ❑ Tomatoes (cherry, Roma, heirloom)
- ❑ Zucchini

FRESH HERBS

- ❑ Basil
- ❑ Chives
- ❑ Cilantro
- ❑ Lemongrass
- ❑ Oregano
- ❑ Parsley
- ❑ Rosemary
- ❑ Shiso
- ❑ Thyme

GRAINS

- ❑ Bran crispbread
- ❑ Low-carb pita pockets
- ❑ Popcorn kernels
- ❑ Quinoa
- ❑ Sprouted-grain bread
- ❑ Steel-cut oats

DAIRY ALTERNATIVES

- ❑ Almond milk, unsweetened
- ❑ Coconut milk, unsweetened
- ❑ Soy creamer, unsweetened
- ❑ Soy yogurt, unsweetened
- ❑ Vegan butter

PROTEINS

- ❑ Almond butter
- ❑ Dry-roasted peanuts, unsalted
- ❑ Low-sodium black beans
- ❑ Low-sodium canned lentils
- ❑ Low-sodium cannellini beans
- ❑ Low-sodium garbanzo beans (chickpeas)
- ❑ Low-sodium red kidney beans
- ❑ Protein powder
- ❑ Raw almonds
- ❑ Raw cashews
- ❑ Red lentils
- ❑ Seitan
- ❑ Slivered almonds
- ❑ Tempeh (smoked)
- ❑ Tofu (extra-firm, silken)

GROCERY

- ❑ Almond flour
- ❑ Almond meal
- ❑ Bamboo shoots
- ❑ Chia seeds
- ❑ Chipotle chiles in adobe sauce
- ❑ Chocolate chunks
- ❑ Cacao nibs
- ❑ Dried seaweed
- ❑ Flaxseeds
- ❑ Goji berries
- ❑ Harissa
- ❑ Kimchi
- ❑ Low-sodium V8 juice
- ❑ Matcha powder
- ❑ Peaches, frozen
- ❑ Roasted red peppers
- ❑ San Marzano tomatoes
- ❑ Unsweetened shredded coconut
- ❑ Vegan mayonnaise
- ❑ Vegetable stock
- ❑ Whole wheat bread crumbs
- ❑ Za'atar

Week 4 Shopping List

PRODUCE

- ❑ Apples (green, Gala)
- ❑ Arugula
- ❑ Asian pears
- ❑ Avocados
- ❑ Bananas
- ❑ Bell pepper (red, green)
- ❑ Blueberries
- ❑ Broccoli
- ❑ Butter lettuce
- ❑ Carrot
- ❑ Cauliflower
- ❑ Celery
- ❑ Clementines
- ❑ Cucumber (English, Japanese)
- ❑ Dates
- ❑ Dried figs
- ❑ Eggplant
- ❑ Garlic
- ❑ Ginger
- ❑ Jalapeño chiles
- ❑ Kale (dinosaur, Tuscan, baby)
- ❑ Kiwis
- ❑ Leeks
- ❑ Lemons
- ❑ Limes
- ❑ Mushroom (cremini, portobello, shiitake)
- ❑ Onions (red, yellow)
- ❑ Oranges
- ❑ Pears
- ❑ Pomegranate arils
- ❑ Raspberries
- ❑ Romaine lettuce
- ❑ Scallion
- ❑ Serrano chiles
- ❑ Shallots
- ❑ Snow peas
- ❑ Spinach
- ❑ Strawberries
- ❑ Sweet potatoes
- ❑ Swiss chard
- ❑ Tomatoes (cherry, Roma, heirloom)
- ❑ Zucchini

FRESH HERBS

- ❑ Basil
- ❑ Cilantro
- ❑ Dill
- ❑ Lemongrass
- ❑ Oregano
- ❑ Parsley
- ❑ Rosemary
- ❑ Thyme

GRAINS

- ❑ Bran crispbread
- ❑ Low-carb pita pockets
- ❑ Quinoa
- ❑ Rolled oats
- ❑ Sprouted-grain bread
- ❑ Sprouted-grain tortillas
- ❑ Steel-cut oats

DAIRY ALTERNATIVES

- ❑ Almond milk yogurt, plain
- ❑ Almond milk, unsweetened
- ❑ Coconut milk, unsweetened
- ❑ Hazelnut milk, unsweetened
- ❑ Soy milk, unsweetened
- ❑ Soy yogurt, unsweetened

PROTEINS

- ❑ Almond butter
- ❑ Dry-roasted peanuts, unsalted
- ❑ Low-sodium black beans
- ❑ Low-sodium canned lentils
- ❑ Low-sodium garbanzo beans (chickpeas)
- ❑ Low-sodium pinto beans
- ❑ Peanut butter (all-natural)
- ❑ Pistachios, unsalted
- ❑ Raw almonds

(continued)

- ❑ Raw cashews
- ❑ Seitan
- ❑ Slivered almonds
- ❑ Tempeh
- ❑ Tofu (extra-firm, silken)
- ❑ Vegan protein powder

- ❑ Chia seeds
- ❑ Dried mulberries
- ❑ Dried seaweed
- ❑ Flaxseeds
- ❑ Garbanzo bean flour
- ❑ Matcha powder
- ❑ Panko bread crumbs
- ❑ Peaches, frozen
- ❑ Pistachios, unsalted
- ❑ Pumpkin puree
- ❑ Pumpkin seeds
- ❑ Roasted red peppers

GROCERY

- ❑ Açai, frozen
- ❑ Almond flour
- ❑ Almond meal
- ❑ Bamboo shoots
- ❑ Cacao nibs
- ❑ Capers

What to Do if You Can't Cook Every Meal at Home?

Don't worry! Here are some easy swaps that you can enjoy if you are on the go.

BREAKFAST CHOICES AWAY FROM HOME

1. Oatmeal: top with berries, cinnamon and nuts
2. Whole-grain toast with peanut butter
3. Smoothie: one serving of fruit with unsweetened almond milk
4. English muffin with peanut butter
5. Unsweetened almond or soy milk yogurt with berries

LUNCH CHOICES AWAY FROM HOME

1. Large Greek salad (omit the feta cheese) topped with falafel
2. Asian stir-fry with tofu
3. Bowl of three-bean chili and a green salad with olive oil and vinegar
4. Chinese: broccoli with bean curd with a small brown rice on the side (use half)
5. Indian: spicy chana masala
6. Mexican: vegetarian fajita (one corn tortilla, no rice, black beans)
7. Italian: arugula salad with a bowl of escarole and bean soup
8. Salad bar: all the vegetables you want!
9. Veggie and hummus sandwich: Whole-grain bread, lettuce, tomato, cucumber, two slices of avocado, sliced carrots and sprouts
10. Lentil soup and a green salad

DINNER CHOICES AWAY FROM HOME

1. Japanese: miso soup, green salad with ginger dressing, two vegetable sushi rolls (preferably made with brown rice)

2. Italian: tricolore salad with eggplant Parmesan (ask them to make it without cheese)

3. Indian: chana masala with 1 cup (144 g) of brown rice and a side of cauliflower

4. Mexican: vegetable tacos with guacamole and salsa and a side of black beans

5. Chinese: mixed vegetables with tofu with a small brown rice

6. Diner: large green salad with a bowl of lentil or vegetable soup with a side of sautéed spinach

7. Veggie burger (no bun) with a small sweet potato with sautéed broccoli

SNACKS ON THE GO

1. Nuts: almonds, walnuts, pistachios

2. Fruit

3. Unsweetened almond or soy yogurt

4. One slice whole-grain bread with peanut or almond butter

5. Hummus and veggies

6. Bowl of vegetable soup

7. 3 crispbreads with sliced avocado

8. Smoothie: one serving of fruit blended with unsweetened almond milk

9. Guacamole and veggies

10. Homemade energy bars (page 93)

To-Do List

❑ Follow the 28-Day Meal Plan.

CHAPTER 7

BREAKFAST

Most people who are trying to lose weight or control their blood sugar have the most difficult time finding healthy selections at breakfast, mostly because the available breakfast choices are laden with calories, fat and sugar. I'm talking about bagels, croissants, donuts and even many yogurts available on the market.

That doesn't have to be the case. With these delicious and easy-to-prepare breakfast choices, you will be out of the house in no time and feeling satisfied. Instead of a bagel with cream cheese, try our Lemon Avocado Toast (page 84) for a satisfying and nutritious blend of carbs and healthy fat. If you don't like avocado, you can top the toast with our Cashew Dream Cheese (page 171). Instead of buying a commercially prepared yogurt, try our Perfect Almond Berry Parfait (page 86)—it has half the calories and carbs of a store-bought version and tastes better! Or if you are in a real rush, instead of grabbing one of those "nutrition" bars (essentially, they are candy bars), prepare our Morning Warrior Bars (page 93) one night during the week or on the weekend, and they will be handy for you to be ready to battle your day!

STRAWBERRY–ALMOND BUTTER PANCAKES

SERVINGS: 2 (FOUR 6″ [15-CM] PANCAKES EACH)

Almond butter (along with other types of nut butters) has recently seen an increase in popularity, providing an alternative to peanut butter. It is lighter in flavor, higher in fiber and lends a lower-carbohydrate substitute to these fluffy pancakes. The strawberries and cinnamon provide just the right amount of sweetness, so you won't even miss the maple syrup. Whip up a batch on the weekend and invite some friends over for brunch.

¼ cup (34 g) almond butter

¼ cup (60 ml) unsweetened almond milk

¼ cup (34 g) silken tofu, blended

¼ tsp baking soda

1 tsp (3 g) ground flaxseeds

1 tsp (3 g) unsweetened shredded coconut

Pinch of salt

Pinch of ground cinnamon

2 tsp (10 ml) coconut oil

½ cup (75 g) sliced strawberries

Thoroughly mix together the almond butter, almond milk, tofu, baking soda, flaxseeds, coconut, salt and cinnamon to combine. The batter should be a pourable consistency (like regular pancake batter).

On a griddle or nonstick pan, heat the coconut oil over medium heat until glistening.

Pour the batter into the center of the pan, continuing to pour directly into the center to keep the pancakes round (the batter will spread naturally) until you have a 6-inch (15-cm) pancake. Top with 4 or 5 slices of strawberry. Cook for 1 to 2 minutes, until golden brown and flip over, cooking for another 1 to 2 minutes on the other side. Continue with the remaining batter. Serve strawberry side up.

NUTRITIONAL INFORMATION PER SERVING: Calories: 325, Total Fat: 25.3 g, Saturated Fat: 7.1 g, Total Carbohydrates: 12.5 g, Fiber: 4.8 g, Net Carbohydrates: 7.7 g, Sugar 4.8 g, Protein: 12.1 g, Sodium: 54.1 mg

LEMON AVOCADO TOAST

SERVINGS: 1

There is an uncomplicated beauty to these toast slices: the creaminess of the avocado, the zing of the lemon and the burst of the tomato all harmonize so well in a recipe that takes less than five minutes to put together. Although this recipe requires only a few ingredients and very little time and effort, it is quite versatile: it creates a fantastic breakfast, go-to snack for when you're in a rush or a great midday meal when served alongside a green salad. You can feel free to make substitutions: Leave off the tomato, add slices of red onion or add sliced radishes and sprinkle with sesame seeds or 1 teaspoon (3 g) of ground flaxseeds.

1 slice sprouted-grain bread
(e.g., Ezekiel brand)

½ avocado, mashed

¼ lemon (wedge)

Pinch of salt

Pinch of black pepper

Pinch of red pepper flakes (optional)

1 slice Roma tomato

Toast the bread to your desired level of brownness. Using a spoon, spread the avocado over the toast. Squeeze the lemon wedge over a small strainer onto the avocado. Sprinkle with the salt, black pepper and red pepper flakes, if using. Top with the tomato slice and enjoy!

NUTRITIONAL INFORMATION PER SERVING: Calories: 198, Total Fat: 7.8 g, Saturated Fat: 0.8 g, Total Carbohydrates: 26.2 g, Fiber: 8.5 g, Net Carbohydrates: 17.7 g, Sugar 6 g, Protein: 6.8 g, Sodium: 182 mg

ENERGIZING AÇAI BOWL

SERVINGS: 1

Açai berries are an antioxidant-packed superfood from Brazil that are as healthy as they are delicious. The puree that serves as the base of this açai bowl is simply a very thick smoothie—meant to be eaten with a spoon. Arrange the toppings over the puree in a pattern, to add a bright and colorful start to your day! Feel free to top with different kinds of fruits on different days to add variety.

1 (3.5 oz [100 g]) packet frozen açai (e.g., Sambazon brand)

¼ cup (60 ml) unsweetened almond milk

½ small banana

¼ cup (34 g) sliced strawberries

¼ cup (34 g) blueberries

1 small kiwi, peeled and sliced

1 tsp (3 g) coconut flakes

1 tsp (3 g) ground flaxseeds

1 tsp (3 g) almond slivers

Break the frozen açai into large chunks within the bag.

Puree the açai with the almond milk and banana until smooth.

Pour the mixture into a chilled glass or bowl and top with the strawberries, blueberries, kiwi, coconut, flaxseeds and almond slivers.

NUTRITIONAL INFORMATION PER SERVING: Calories: 290, Total Fat: 10.6 g, Saturated Fat: 2.2 g, Total Carbohydrates: 41.5 g, Fiber: 11.7 g, Net Carbohydrates: 29.8 g, Sugar 24.4 g, Protein: 5.6 g, Sodium: 65.8 mg

PERFECT ALMOND BERRY PARFAIT

SERVINGS: 2

Almond yogurt is a wonderful product that takes advantage of the versatility of almonds to create a fantastic substitute for yogurt in a plant-based diet. These breakfast treats look especially beautiful when the fruit, yogurt and granola are layered in glass stemware. Top with 1 teaspoon (3 g) of ground flaxseed if you have it in the house.

6 oz (170 g) plain almond yogurt

¼ cup (34 g) sliced banana

¼ cup (34 g) sliced strawberries

¼ cup (34) blueberries

¼ cup (34 g) Granola Clusters (page 142)

In a parfait glass, start with a layer of almond yogurt. Add one-third of the banana slices, one-third of the strawberries, one-third of the blueberries and one-third of the homemade granola.

Add another layer of almond yogurt. Follow with another layer of fruit and granola.

Repeat with a final layer of yogurt and fruit and granola.

NUTRITIONAL INFORMATION PER SERVING: Calories: 165, Total Fat: 5.1 g, Saturated Fat: 0.5 g, Total Carbohydrates: 27.6 g, Fiber: 3.3 g, Net Carbohydrates: 24.3 g, Sugar 13.1 g, Protein: 3.3 g, Sodium: 33.2 mg

BERRY BLISS SMOOTHIE

SERVINGS: 1

Smoothies are an excellent way to integrate a more nutritious diet with an on-the-go lifestyle. If you are able to get fresh berries, the result is delicious, but frozen berries are an excellent choice, too; you can stock up without having to worry about cost or perishability. Additionally, you can premeasure all of the frozen ingredients for a week's worth of smoothies at once and keep each serving in a plastic sandwich bag in the freezer. Smoothies are a great meal replacement when made at home, but be careful when ordering smoothies out—many are laden with sugar and calories.

8 oz (220 ml) unsweetened almond milk

¼ tsp matcha powder

1 tbsp (9 g) flaxseeds

¼ cup (34 g) raspberries

¼ cup (34 g) blueberries

¼ cup (34 g) roughly chopped strawberries, plus one slice (optional)

3 ice cubes

3 oz (85 g) silken tofu (optional—for thicker smoothie)

Puree all the ingredients together until smooth. Garnish with an extra slice of strawberry, if desired.

You can substitute frozen fruit—just omit the ice cubes.

NUTRITIONAL INFORMATION PER SERVING: Calories: 200, Total Fat: 8.7 g, Saturated Fat: 0.4 g, Total Carbohydrates: 19.5 g, Fiber: 7.6 g, Net Carbohydrates: 11.9 g, Sugar 13.9 g, Protein: 10 g, Sodium: 149.3 mg

GREEN GODDESS SMOOTHIE

SERVINGS: 1

Spinach is an extremely versatile food that serves as an excellent staple in any diet. The bright green color of this smoothie can be deceiving—it tastes as if it's packed with nothing but sweet, delicious fruit. Choosing a vanilla-flavored protein powder further enhances these flavors, for a produce-filled breakfast that tastes like dessert! Try substituting Swiss chard or romaine lettuce if you don't have spinach in the house.

1 cup (136 g) fresh spinach, packed tightly

½ cup (68 g) frozen peaches

1 small banana

1 cup (237 ml) unsweetened almond milk

1 scoop favorite protein powder or vegetable powder (optional)

4 ice cubes, if using fresh peaches

Combine all the ingredients in a blender and blend until very smooth.

NUTRITIONAL INFORMATION PER SERVING: Calories: 295, Total Fat: 3.7 g, Saturated Fat: 0.6 g, Total Carbohydrates: 46 g, Fiber: 7 g, Net Carbohydrates: 39 g, Sugar 27.5 g, Protein: 11.2 g, Sodium: 217.2 mg

GLOWING GREEN SMOOTHIE

SERVINGS: 2

This smoothie is ideal for mornings when you're craving something bright and crisp, rather than sweet and indulgent. The addition of the apples and limes in this smoothie make it just as flavorful and delicious as fruit-filled alternatives.

1 cup (136 g) chopped dinosaur kale, packed tightly

1 cup (136 g) fresh spinach, packed tightly

½ cup (68 g) julienned cucumber

½ cup (68 g) chopped celery

Juice of ½ lime

1 cup (236 ml) water

½ cup (68 g) cored and chopped Fuji apple

4 ice cubes

Combine all the ingredients in a blender and blend until very smooth.

NUTRITIONAL INFORMATION PER SERVING: Calories: 80, Total Fat: 0.5 g, Saturated Fat: 0.1 g, Total Carbohydrates: 15 g, Fiber: 2.6 g, Net Carbohydrates: 12.4 g, Sugar 2 g, Protein: 2.3 g, Sodium: 45.4 mg

SPICED STEEL-CUT OATS

SERVINGS: 4

Steel-cut oats are a nutrition powerhouse that are a satisfying and filling way to start your day. Since they take longer to digest than rolled oats do, they produce less of an insulin response, which is important when you are trying to lower your A1c. This recipe calls for quick-cooking oats in the interest of saving time; however, you can buy original steel-cut oats (which take about 30 minutes to make) and make up a batch on the weekends; just reheat during the week.

¾ cup (177 ml) water

¼ cup (40 g) quick-cooking steel-cut oatmeal (e.g., Bob's Red Mill brand)

¼ cup (60 ml) unsweetened almond milk

½ tsp pumpkin pie spice

1 tsp (3 g) dried currants or raisins (optional)

2 tsp (3 g) unsweetened shredded coconut, toasted (optional)

¼ cup (34 g) blueberries (optional)

Bring the water to a rolling boil in a small saucepot.

Add the oats and lower the heat to medium-low. Cook for 7 minutes, stirring constantly. Turn off the heat.

Add the almond milk and pumpkin pie spice. Stir to combine.

Serve with the currants, coconut and blueberries, if desired.

NUTRITIONAL INFORMATION PER SERVING: Calories: 100, Total Fat: 2.5 g, Saturated Fat: 1.1 g, Total Carbohydrates: 17.7 g, Fiber: 2.7 g, Net Carbohydrates: 15 g, Sugar 8.2 g, Protein: 2.5 g, Sodium: 43.5 mg

SUNNY SCRAMBLED TOFU WITH MARKET VEGETABLES

SERVINGS: 2

Rise and shine with this delicious veggie scramble. Start off your day on the right foot by fueling up with this yummy meal. The protein in the tofu will stabilize your blood sugar throughout the day, and the fiber-packed veggies will keep you full, not to mention give you a big boost of phytonutrients, so you're ready to take on whatever the day throws at you.

2 tsp (10 ml) sesame oil

1 (14 oz [397 g]) block extra-firm tofu, cubed

2 scallions, sliced

¼ tsp minced garlic

4 oz (113 g) shiitake or oyster mushrooms, sliced

1 red bell pepper, chopped

4 oz (113 g) broccoli florets, cut very small

Pinch of ground cumin

Pinch of black pepper

Pinch of red chili flakes (optional)

In a nonstick pan, heat 1 teaspoon (5 ml) of the sesame oil over high heat until the pan is shiny. Add the tofu cubes in an even layer and sear on each side until golden brown. Transfer the tofu to a bowl.

Add the remaining 1 teaspoon (5 ml) of the sesame oil to the pan and heat until the pan is shiny. Add the scallions, garlic, mushrooms, bell pepper, broccoli, cumin, black pepper and red chili flakes, if using. Sauté for 3 to 4 minutes.

Add the tofu back to the pan and stir to combine, being careful not to break up the tofu cubes.

NUTRITIONAL INFORMATION PER SERVING: Calories: 287, Total Fat: 15 g, Saturated Fat: 2 g, Carbohydrates: 16 g, Fiber: 5 g, Net Carbohydrates: 11 g, Sugar: 4 g, Protein: 24 g, Sodium: 215 mg

EXTREMELY TASTY VEGETABLE "FRITTATA"

SERVINGS: 4

This cholesterol-free alternative to a classic breakfast favorite is sure to be a hit at brunch. The baking powder gives the tofu the same airy, fluffy quality of eggs, and adding in a rainbow of vegetables will brighten up anyone's morning. Serve it as is or accompany with 1 cup (136 g) of berries or a slice of sprouted-grain toast.

1 (3.5 oz [28 g]) block soft silken tofu

3 tbsp (28 g) cornstarch

1 tsp (4 g) baking powder

1 tsp (5 g) salt plus a pinch

1 tbsp (115 ml) extra-virgin olive oil

4 oz (113 g) yellow onion, diced

4 oz (113 g) red bell pepper, diced

1 jalapeño chile, seeded and sliced

4 oz (113 g) cremini mushrooms, sliced

4 oz (113 g) chopped asparagus

Pinch of black pepper

Preheat the oven to broil. Using a blender (the mixture is wet and a food processor might leak), puree the tofu, cornstarch, baking powder and 1 teaspoon (5 g) of salt until fully combined. Set aside.

Heat the extra-virgin olive oil in a medium rondeau or sauté pan over medium heat until the oil glistens. Add the onion and sauté for 1 minute.

Add the rest of the vegetables and sauté for another 4 to 5 minutes.

Stir in the tofu mixture to combine thoroughly with rest of vegetables and smooth out the top. Continue to cook for 10 minutes.

Put the pan in the oven and broil for 1 to 2 minutes, until the top is golden brown. Sprinkle with a pinch of salt and the black pepper.

Remove the frittata from the pan and let rest for 5 minutes prior to serving.

NUTRITIONAL INFORMATION PER SERVING: Calories: 104, Total Fat: 3.7 g, Saturated Fat: 0.3 g, Total Carbohydrates: 12.6 g, Fiber: 2.1 g, Net Carbohydrates: 10.5 g, Sugar 3.6 g, Protein: 3.9 g, Sodium: 92 mg

MORNING WARRIOR BARS

SERVINGS: 8

These bars are delicious and versatile. You can eat them in the morning for breakfast, accompanied by almond yogurt, or on their own before a workout or as a snack accompanied by a fruit in the afternoon. They are high in fiber and low in sugar. Many of the commercial bars on the market are essentially glorified candy bars—high in calories and loaded with sugar. These homemade bars are easy to make and delicious.

4 oz (113 g) dates, pitted

¼ cup (19 g) unsweetened shredded coconut

¾ cup (128 g) raw almonds

¾ cup (83 g) raw cashews

½ tsp pumpkin pie spice

1 tsp (3 g) flaxseeds

2 tbsp (30 ml) coconut oil (should be solid, not liquid)

In a food processor, process the dates until a ball begins to form. Add the coconut, almonds and cashews. Process until the mixture is fine and crumbly.

Add the pumpkin pie spice and flaxseeds. Process to mix thoroughly.

Add the coconut oil and process until the mixture resembles a sticky dough.

Scoop into small balls. Alternatively, transfer the entire mixture to a sheet of waxed paper and roll out into a square, then use a lightly oiled knife to cut out 8 equal bars.

NUTRITIONAL INFORMATION PER SERVING: Calories: 260, Total Fat: 20 g, Saturated Fat: 5 g, Carbohydrates: 18 g, Fiber: 3 g, Net Carbohydrates: 15 g, Sugar: 10 g, Protein: 7 g, Sodium: 5 mg

CHIA SEED PUDDING

SERVINGS: 4

Chia seeds are so interesting because when they are combined with a liquid, the seeds begin to form a gel, which will give the mixture a pudding-like consistency in a matter of hours. This thick consistency keeps you fuller longer and helps stabilize your blood sugar. The result is an extremely versatile food that you can add almost any fruit to—this recipe suggests antioxidant-rich pomegranate and blueberries, to give you an extra boost.

1 cup (236 ml) unsweetened coconut milk

6 oz (170 g) unsweetened soy yogurt

¼ cup (40 g) chia seeds

¼ cup (34 g) pomegranate arils

¼ cup (34 g) blueberries

1 tbsp (9 g) almond slivers (optional)

Whisk together the coconut milk, soy yogurt and chia seeds in a small bowl.

Cover with plastic wrap and refrigerate for a minimum of 4 hours, preferably overnight.

Top with the pomegranate arils, blueberries and almonds, if using.

NUTRITIONAL INFORMATION PER SERVING: Calories: 251, Total Fat: 16.8 g, Saturated Fat: 9.8 g, Total Carbohydrates: 17.6 g, Fiber: 7.2 g, Net Carbohydrates: 10.4 g, Sugar 8.9 g, Protein: 7.6 g, Sodium: 54.4 mg

VEGAN PUMPKIN MUFFINS

YIELDS 12 MUFFINS; SERVING SIZE: 1 MUFFIN

These muffins have so much texture and flavor, no one will ever know they lack butter and eggs. Pumpkin puree is one of my favorite ingredients as it is full of fiber, vitamin C and beta-carotene and is now readily available in grocery stores all year long. This sweet treat is so tasty, it's hard to believe it's good for you! Try one alongside a veggie-packed omelet for a balanced breakfast. They also make a great dessert or the perfect midday snack. Try doubling the recipe and freezing extras, so you always have a few on hand.

1 tbsp (9 g) flaxseed meal + 2 tbsp (30 ml) water, mixed well

¾ cup (177 ml) unsweetened hazelnut milk

1 tsp (5 ml) vanilla extract

2 tbsp (30 ml) hazelnut oil

2 tbsp (30 ml) pure maple syrup

½ cup (68 g) pure pumpkin puree

¾ cup (94 g) all-purpose flour

¼ tsp (6 g) baking soda

1½ tsp (6 g) baking powder

¼ tsp salt

¼ cup (50 g) golden brown sugar

¼ cup (25 g) almond meal

1 tbsp (10 g) pumpkin seeds

Preheat the oven to 375°F (190°C). Grease a cupcake or muffin pan, or line with liners, if desired.

Combine the flaxseed mixture, hazelnut milk, vanilla extract, hazelnut oil, maple syrup and pumpkin puree.

In a separate bowl, whisk together the flour, baking soda, baking powder, salt, brown sugar and almond meal.

Stir the dry ingredients into the wet ingredients until thoroughly combined.

Fill the prepared cupcake wells three-quarters of the way to the top. Sprinkle the batter with the pumpkin seeds.

Bake for 45 to 60 minutes, or until the muffins spring back when pushed gently.

Let cool for 10 minutes.

NUTRITION INFORMATION PER SERVING: Calories: 107, Total Fat: 4 g, Saturated Fat: 0 g, Total Carbohydrates: 16 g, Fiber: 1 g, Net Carbohydrates: 15 g, Sugar: 8 g, Protein: 2 g, Sodium: 146 mg

CHAPTER 8

LUNCH

Lunch is one of my favorite meals and soon it will be one of yours! Gone are the days of mundane sandwiches and boring salads. You might think that you have no time to eat—or only enough time to grab a quick bite at the drive-through or to scarf something down at the office—but with just a little planning, you can have scrumptious meals for the whole week. Whether you are eating at your desk, staying home with your kids or enjoying a leisurely lunch with friends or family, these recipes have you covered.

For a tantalizing meal that takes minutes to make, try the Portobello Kimchi Lettuce Wraps (page 105); or if you're feeling "saucy," enjoy the Spicy Tempeh Salad (page 113); or if you do feel like having a sandwich, go for a new version of an old classic—the BLT—the Guiltless Seitan "BLT" Pockets (page 109).

The lunches provided here have a healthy, balanced combination of all the nutrients your body needs to get you through the afternoon with enough energy until dinnertime. These easy-to-prepare recipes contain a tasty combination of carbohydrates, satisfying fiber, lean protein and healthy fats. Not only are they delicious, they are also nutritious.

SOUTHWESTERN SALAD

SERVINGS: 2

Spice things up with this delicious Southwestern salad. Chock-full of protein, thanks to yummy black beans, it's sure to keep you full and enable you to maintain a healthy blood sugar all day long. Plus the perfect combination of flavors will leave you satisfied; the creaminess of the avocados and the sweetness of the tomatoes pair superbly with the zesty jalapeño lime dressing.

4 oz (113 g) precooked tempeh, cut into ½" (1.9 cm) cubes

Salt and black pepper

1 cup (136 g) canned or cooked black beans

½ avocado, sliced lengthwise

8 cherry tomatoes, halved

4 thin rings red onion

1 cup (136 g) baby kale

¼ cup (34 g) chopped roasted red pepper

1 tbsp (9 g) chopped fresh cilantro

JALAPEÑO LIME DRESSING

1 tbsp (15 ml) extra-virgin olive oil

Juice of 1 lime

2 tsp (11 ml) whole-grain mustard

1 small jalapeño chile, seeded, deveined and minced

1 tbsp (9 g) chopped fresh cilantro

1 tbsp (9 ml) honey

Salt and black pepper

Season both sides of the cubed tempeh with the salt and pepper.

Generously coat a skillet with oil. Heat over medium heat until shiny. Brown the tempeh on all sides, 1 to 2 minutes per side.

Make the dressing: In a bowl, whisk together the extra-virgin olive oil, lime juice, mustard, jalapeño, cilantro, honey and salt and pepper to taste.

Put the rest of the salad ingredients in the bowl and drizzle with the prepared dressing. Toss to coat. Add more salt and pepper to taste.

NUTRITIONAL INFORMATION PER SERVING:
SALAD: Calories: 270, Total Fat: 8 g, Saturated Fat: 1 g, Total Carbohydrates: 38 g, Fiber: 31 g, Net Carbohydrates: 25 g, Sugar: 4 g, Protein: 12 g, Sodium: 310 mg
DRESSING: Calories: 110, Total Fat: 7 g, Saturated Fat: 1 g, Total Carbohydrates: 10 g, Fiber: 0 g, Net Carbohydrates: 10 g, Sugar: 9 g, Protein: 0 g, Sodium: 120 mg

ARUGULA AND WILD MUSHROOM SALAD WITH CITRUS-WALNUT DRESSING

SERVINGS: 2

This refreshing salad is full of vitamins, minerals and fiber. Choosing walnut oil not only adds a nutty flavor to the peppery arugula leaves, but gives you a boost of heart-healthy omega-3 fatty acids. Enjoy with a warm bowl of vegetable soup for a satisfying lunch or dinner. Add a handful of pomegranate arils and chopped walnuts, if you have them in the house—they will make a great addition.

¼ cup (34 g) extra-firm tofu

2 cups (272 g) arugula leaves

½ cup (68 g) cherry tomatoes, halved

½ cup (68 g) thinly sliced cremini mushrooms

¼ cup (34 g) canned or cooked pinto beans

1 tsp (5 ml) lemon juice

1 tbsp (15 ml) walnut oil

½ tsp Dijon mustard

⅛ tsp salt

Black pepper

Drain the tofu and remove any excess water by placing the tofu between paper towels and resting a bowl on top for 5 minutes. This will press out the liquid.

Cut the tofu into small squares.

Place the arugula in a large bowl and add the tofu, tomatoes, mushrooms and pinto beans.

Add the lemon juice, walnut oil, mustard, salt and pepper to taste. Toss and serve.

NUTRITIONAL INFORMATION PER SERVING: Calories: 153, Total Fat: 10 g, Saturated Fat: 1 g, Total Carbohydrates: 10 g, Fiber: 4 g, Net Carbohydrates: 6 g, Sugar: 2 g, Protein: 8 g, Sodium: 162 mg

CURLY KALE SALAD

SERVINGS: 2

All of the vibrant colors in this salad make it a beautiful addition to any table! The avocado in this dressing makes it wonderfully creamy and is the perfect substitute for rich, fatty salad dressings. Kale is a great alternative to other more traditional lettuces that you are used to seeing in salads—variety is the spice of life!

DRESSING

½ avocado, pitted and peeled

1 clove garlic

2 tbsp (30 ml) extra-virgin olive oil

3 tbsp (44 ml) lime juice

Salt and black pepper

½ cup (68 g) uncooked multicolored quinoa

1 cup (237 ml) water

8 oz (227 g) curly kale, torn into bite-size pieces

1 yellow bell pepper, julienned

8 thinly mandolined rings red onion, halved

Make the dressing: Puree all the dressing ingredients together, adding salt and black pepper to taste.

Place the quinoa and water in a small stockpot. Bring to a boil. Lower the heat, cover and simmer for about 10 minutes. Once the water evaporates, remove from the heat and let cool.

Toss the dressing with the quinoa, kale, bell pepper and onion until well combined.

NUTRITIONAL INFORMATION PER SERVING: Calories: 331, Total Fat: 23.8 g, Saturated Fat: 3.1 g, Total Carbohydrates: 22.9 g, Fiber: 9.2 g, Net Carbohydrates: 13.7 g, Sugar: 2.4 g, Protein: 8 g, Sodium: 90 mg

ZESTY TOMATO AND AVOCADO TARTINE

SERVINGS: 2 SLICES

Avocados are the greatest thing to happen to bread since slicing it. When ripe, avocados can be mashed to the perfect, smooth consistency and will spread right on your slice of sprouted-grain bread. Top it with thinly sliced Roma tomatoes, some whole-grain mustard and a squeeze of lime juice, and your taste buds are sure to be dancing.

½ avocado, mashed

½ tsp flaxseeds

1 tsp (5 ml) whole-grain mustard

1 tsp (5 ml) lime juice

2 slices sprouted-grain bread (e.g., Ezekiel brand), toasted

2 thin slices Roma tomato

6 leaves arugula

Salt and black pepper

Mix together the avocado, flaxseeds, mustard and lime juice. Spread on the toasted bread.

Top with the tomato and arugula. Add salt and pepper to taste.

NUTRITIONAL INFORMATION PER SERVING (without bread): Calories: 90, Total Fat: 8 g, Saturated Fat: 1 g, Total Carbohydrates: 6 g, Fiber: 4 g, Net Carbohydrates: 2 g, Sugar: 3 g, Protein: 1 g, Sodium: 160 mg

AUTUMN HARVEST CHICKPEA SALAD

SERVINGS: 1

Garbanzo beans and celery are both very mild and delicate tasting on their own. In this salad, they are combined with flavor-packed capers, dill and lemon, so you get all of the nutritional benefit of the beans and celery in a salad that tastes delicious.

1 cup (136 g) canned garbanzo beans (chickpeas), drained and rinsed

1 medium rib celery, diced

2 tsp (6 g) capers

1 or 2 sprigs dill, chopped

Juice of ½ lemon

1½ tsp (7 ml) extra-virgin olive oil

Salt

Black pepper

Red pepper flakes (optional)

Combine all the ingredients in a bowl, adding salt, black pepper and red pepper flakes, if desired, to taste.

Let sit in the fridge for 1 hour to combine the flavors.

Enjoy!

NUTRITIONAL INFORMATION PER SERVING: Calories: 176, Total Fat: 8.8 g, Saturated Fat: 0.9 g, Total Carbohydrates: 21.8 g, Fiber: 5.7 g, Net Carbohydrates: 16.1 g, Sugar 2.5 g, Protein: 5.6 g, Sodium: 200 mg

MINI BAKED FALAFEL BURGERS IN LETTUCE CUPS WITH CUCUMBER-YOGURT SAUCE

YIELD: 8 FALAFEL BALLS AND 1 CUP (237 ML) OF SAUCE; SERVINGS: 2

Traditional falafel is deep-fried and laden with extra calories and fat. Finishing baked falafel under the broiler provides a crunchy exterior while leaving the inside nice and fluffy. Turmeric not only adds a beautiful color to the dish, but has been shown to have anti-inflammatory and antioxidant effects on the body. Two lettuce wraps and a side salad make the perfect Middle Eastern–inspired meal. You have the option to serve with an Israeli Salad (page 153) or a bowl of cucumber soup.

FALAFEL

3 tbsp (45 ml) extra-virgin olive oil

1 (15 oz [425 g]) can garbanzo beans (chickpeas), drained and rinsed

½ cup (68 g) diced red onion

2 small cloves garlic

½ cup (68 g) garbanzo bean flour

3 tbsp (26 g) chopped fresh parsley

2 tsp (6 g) ground cumin

¼ tsp ground turmeric

1 tsp (3 g) salt

½ tsp black pepper

CUCUMBER YOGURT SAUCE

½ cup (68 g) plain nonfat soy yogurt

½ small cucumber, chopped

1 tbsp (9 g) chopped fresh parsley

1 tbsp (15 ml) lemon juice

½ tsp salt

8 pieces butter leaf lettuce, to serve

Preheat the oven to 375°F (190°C). Line a baking sheet with aluminum foil. Lightly spray with extra-virgin olive oil.

Make the falafel: Place the falafel ingredients in a food processor. Puree until medium chunky.

Shape the mixture into medium balls and place on the prepared baking sheet. Bake for 20 to 25 minutes.

As they are baking, make the dressing. Combine the dressing ingredients and puree until smooth. Chill in the refrigerator.

Once the falafel balls are done baking, change the oven setting to broil and broil the falafel for 3 minutes. Remove from the oven and let cool.

Serve the falafel balls in the butter leaf lettuce and top with the cucumber yogurt sauce.

NUTRITIONAL INFORMATION PER SERVING: Calories: 131, Total Fat: 7 g, Saturated Fat: 1 g, Total Carbohydrates: 13 g, Fiber: 3 g, Net Carbohydrates: 10 g, Sugar: 3 g, Protein: 6 g, Sodium: 533 mg

WINTER WHITE BEAN SOUP WITH KALE AND BASIL PISTOU

YIELD: 5 CUPS (1.2 L) OF SOUP AND 1 CUP (136 G) OF PISTOU; SERVINGS: 5

When the weather starts to get a little colder there is nothing more satisfying than a bowl of warm soup. This hearty yet sophisticated soup is both warming and fulfilling. Kale is a fibrous green that holds up well in soups and can withstand multiple rounds of reheating. Its emerald green color packs this super veggie with vitamins A, C and K. A dollop of pistou adds an herbaceous kick while providing a healthy dose of rich, heart-healthy fat. Enjoy with a side salad.

SOUP

2 tbsp (30 ml) extra-virgin olive oil

½ cup (68 g) minced yellow onion

¼ cup (34 g) diced celery

¼ cup (34 g) diced carrot

2 cloves garlic, minced

2 tbsp (30 ml) lemon juice

1 (15 oz [425 g]) can cannellini beans, drained and rinsed

3 cups (710 ml) vegetable stock

1 bunch red Russian kale, stemmed and chopped

Salt and black pepper

PISTOU

1 zucchini, cored and cut into small cubes (cut out a rectangle from the middle so only the green outer edges remain; use the rest to make Vegetable Lasagne with Cashew Ricotta [page 122])

1 clove garlic, sliced

¼ cup (60 ml) extra-virgin olive oil

3 large leaves fresh basil

¼ cup (38 g) nutritional yeast

Juice of ½ lemon

Salt and black pepper

Make the soup: Heat the extra-virgin olive oil in a stockpot over medium heat until shiny. Add the onion, celery, carrot and garlic and cook until fragrant. Deglaze with the lemon juice.

Add the beans and sauté for 1 to 2 minutes. Add the vegetable stock and bring to a light boil. Lower the heat, cover and let simmer for 10 minutes, or until all the vegetables are soft.

Add the kale and cook for another 10 minutes over low heat. Add salt and black pepper to taste.

While the soup is finishing, make the pistou: Sauté the zucchini, garlic and extra-virgin olive oil in a separate large pan over medium heat, until the zucchini is slightly cooked through, about 5 minutes. Add the basil and cook for 1 minute.

In a food processor, puree with the rest of the pistou ingredients until slightly chunky.

Remove the soup from the heat and add salt and pepper to taste. Serve in a bowl with a large dollop of the pistou.

NUTRITIONAL INFORMATION PER SERVING: Calories: 284, Total Fat: 18 g, Saturated Fat: 2 g, Total Carbohydrates: 25 g, Fiber: 7 g, Net Carbohydrates: 18 g, Sugar: 5 g, Protein: 10 g, Sodium: 450 mg

CURRIED TOFU PITA POCKETS

SERVINGS: 4

These pita pockets are a delicious way to impress company. They showcase the wonderful power of greens as they contain several different types of green veggies, all of which contribute a completely unique flavor; from the gentle sweetness of the basil to the strong earthiness of the kale.

1 tbsp (15 ml) extra-virgin olive oil

1 (14 oz [397 g]) block extra-firm tofu, halved and then sliced

1 tbsp (9 g) curry powder

Pinch of cayenne pepper

3 tbsp (26 g) vegan mayonnaise

Juice of ½ lemon

1 tsp (5 g) salt

PER POCKET

1 whole wheat low-carb pita pocket

7 leaves baby kale

1 tbsp (9 g) grated carrot

1 tbsp (9 g) thinly sliced celery

1 tsp (2 g) thinly sliced scallion

2 leaves fresh basil

Heat the extra-virgin olive oil in a sauté pan until slick and shiny.

Sear the tofu for about 30 seconds on each side, until all sides are golden brown. Remove from the heat and set aside.

In a small bowl, combine the curry powder, cayenne, mayonnaise, lemon juice and salt. Mix well.

Toss the curry mixture, 1 tablespoon (9 g) at a time, with the tofu until the tofu is well coated.

Warm the pita pockets in the oven, if desired. Place one-quarter of the tofu mixture inside each pita. Top the tofu with the kale, carrot, celery, scallion and basil.

NUTRITIONAL INFORMATION PER SERVING: Calories: 326, Total Fat: 17.8 g, Saturated Fat: 0.7 g, Total Carbohydrates: 27 g, Fiber: 8.7 g, Net Carbohydrates: 18.3 g, Sugar 0.8 g, Protein: 21 g, Sodium: 402 mg

PORTOBELLO KIMCHI LETTUCE WRAPS

SERVINGS: 4

Kimchi (Korean fermented vegetables) is known for a whole host of health-promoting effects. Its benefits include anticancer, antiobesity, colorectal health promotion, probiotic properties, cholesterol reduction, antioxidative and antiaging properties, brain health promotion, immune promotion and skin health promotion, to name a few. Kimchi can be eaten in a variety of ways, from sautéing it with leafy green vegetables to making it into a stew. One of my favorite ways to enjoy it is to pair it with portobello mushrooms in these tasty lettuce wraps.

1 tbsp (15 ml) extra-virgin olive oil

2 portobello mushrooms, sliced lengthwise and halved

Pinch of salt

Pinch of black pepper

¼ cup (34 g) uncooked quinoa

½ cup (118 ml) water

1 green bell pepper, sliced thinly

1 cup (136 g) kimchi (napa cabbage variety)

4 leaves romaine or butter lettuce

½ avocado, diced

1 tbsp (9 g) thinly sliced scallion

¼ cup (35 g) julienned cucumber

4 cherry tomatoes, halved

In a nonstick pan, heat the extra-virgin olive oil over high heat until shiny. Add the portobello mushrooms, sprinkle with the salt and black pepper and sauté until golden on both sides, 1 to 2 minutes per side. Remove from the pan and set aside.

Place the quinoa and water in a small stockpot. Bring to a boil. Lower the heat, cover and simmer for about 10 minutes. Once the water evaporates, remove from the heat and let cool.

Add the bell pepper and kimchi to the pan and sauté for 3 to 4 minutes over medium heat.

Add the portobello mushrooms back to the pan along with the cooked quinoa and toss to combine over low heat.

Assemble the lettuce wraps by layering on the avocado, portobello mixture, scallion, cucumber and tomatoes.

NUTRITIONAL INFORMATION PER SERVING: Calories: 143, Total Fat: 7 g, Saturated Fat: 1 g, Total Carbohydrates: 16 g, Fiber: 4 g, Net Carbohydrates: 12 g, Sugar: 5 g, Protein: 6 g, Sodium: 550 mg

AVOCADO AND TOMATO SANDWICH

SERVINGS: 1

The creamy consistency of the avocado on this sandwich works just as well as any spread will—think of this sandwich as your new PB&J. The tomato and cucumber provide the perfect crunch, and the Omega Power Bread is an excellent choice of low-carb bread. Overall, this sandwich is the ideal midday treat to keep you happy inside and outside! Add some sprouts or mung beans if you have them in the house—they will add a pop in your mouth. You can also drizzle with a little balsamic vinegar, if you feel like it.

⅓ avocado, sliced

2 slices Healthy Joy Omega Power Bread

½ sliced tomato

½ cucumber, sliced

1 tsp (5 ml) extra-virgin olive oil

Salt and black pepper

Mash the avocado with a fork and spread evenly over the bread.

Layer the tomato and cucumber on top.

Drizzle the extra-virgin olive oil over the tomato and cucumber.

Add salt and black pepper to taste.

NUTRITIONAL INFORMATION PER SERVING: Calories: 321, Total Fat: 19.5 g, Saturated Fat: 2.1 g, Total Carbohydrates: 18.9 g, Fiber: 13.5 g, Net Carbohydrates: 5.4 g, Sugar 3.1 g, Protein: 20.1 g, Sodium: 114 mg

VEGETARIAN QUINOA AND BLACK BEAN WRAPS

SERVINGS: 1 (4 TO 6 WRAPS)

Looking for something to grab in a hurry? A nutritious meal-to-go has never been easier. This wrap is a cinch to throw together, but packs a huge nutritional punch. Quinoa and beans are full of protein and fiber; carrots, cucumbers and oranges provide important vitamins and minerals, and peanut butter is a great source of healthy fats. You can make the peanut sauce a day ahead.

½ cup (68 g) uncooked quinoa

1 cup (237 ml) water

½ cup (68 g) canned or cooked black beans

1 tbsp (9 g) chopped fresh cilantro

¼ cup (34 g) shredded carrot

¼ cup (34 g) shredded cucumber

1 tbsp (9 g) sliced scallion

4 to 6 leaves butter or romaine lettuce

½ orange, segmented

1 tsp (3 g) black sesame seeds

PEANUT BUTTER SOY SAUCE DRESSING

1 tbsp (9 g) peanut butter

1 tsp (5 ml) sesame oil

1 tsp (5 ml) low-sodium soy sauce

1 tbsp (15 ml) lime juice

Place the quinoa and water in a small stockpot. Bring to a boil. Lower the heat, cover and simmer for about 10 minutes. Once the water evaporates, remove from the heat and let cool.

While the quinoa cools, make the dressing: Mix together the peanut butter, sesame oil, soy sauce and lime juice in small bowl. Whisk to combine.

Toss the quinoa, black beans, cilantro, carrot, cucumber and scallion with the dressing.

Place the quinoa mixture on the lettuce leaves and top with the orange segments and black sesame seeds.

NUTRITIONAL INFORMATION PER SERVING:
WRAPS: Calories: 280, Total Fat: 2.5 g, Saturated Fat: 0 g, Total Carbohydrates: 53 g, Fiber: 13 g, Net Carbohydrates: 40 g, Sugar: 1 g, Protein: 13 g, Sodium: 350 mg
DRESSING: Calories: 25, Total Fat: 2.5 g, Saturated Fat: 0 g, Total Carbohydrates: 1 g, Fiber: 0 g, Net Carbohydrates: 1 g, Sugar: 0 g, Protein: 1 g, Sodium: 45 mg

CHICKPEA SOUP

SERVINGS: 3

Some days, there is nothing that can replace a hearty bowl of soup. This recipe has so much flavor and is incredibly warming. The garbanzo beans that serve as the main body of this soup become very smooth and creamy when blended, and the end result is a bowl of soup that is very filling but chock-full of ingredients that are great for you.

6 tbsp (89 ml) olive oil, plus more for garnish (optional)

6 cloves garlic, sliced thinly

½ tsp red pepper flakes, plus more for garnish (optional)

3 (15 oz [425 g]) cans garbanzo beans (chickpeas), drained and rinsed

4 cups (946 ml) vegetable stock

⅛ tsp salt

Drizzle of cider vinegar

Combine 3 tablespoons (45 ml) of the extra-virgin olive oil and the garlic and red pepper flakes in a sauté pan. Cook over medium heat for about 1 minute.

Add the chickpeas and cook for 2 more minutes, stirring occasionally.

Add the vegetable stock and bring to a boil. Lower the heat and simmer for 30 minutes.

Add the remaining 3 tablespoons (45 ml) of the olive oil. Blend until smooth with an immersion blender. Add the salt and the cider vinegar.

Add additional red pepper flakes and a drop of olive oil, if desired.

NUTRITIONAL INFORMATION PER SERVING: Calories: 188, Total Fat: 10 g, Saturated Fat: 1.4 g, Total Carbohydrates: 15.3 g, Fiber: 6.7 g, Net Carbohydrates: 8.7 g, Sugar: 1.2 g, Protein: 6 g, Sodium: 463 mg

GUILTLESS SEITAN "BLT" POCKETS

SERVINGS: 4 POCKETS

Who didn't love a nice BLT while growing up? Luckily, I was able to re-create the childhood delight without all of the saturated fat and empty calories. This seitan "BLT" has the same great taste you know and love, but is also packed with nutrients and high in protein, vitamin C, thiamine, riboflavin, niacin and iron. There's nothing to feel guilty about when indulging in this amazing sandwich.

4 whole wheat pita pockets

8 oz (227 g) seitan, sliced ¼" (6.35-mm) thick, patted dry

Pinch of onion powder

Pinch of garlic powder

Pinch of ground cumin

Pinch of paprika

Pinch of dried thyme

Salt and black pepper

Dash of Worcestershire sauce

1 tbsp (15 ml) extra-virgin olive oil

4 tsp (12 g) vegan mayonnaise

8 leaves romaine lettuce

12 slices Roma tomato

12 thin slices red onion

Chopped fresh cilantro (optional)

Prepared mustard

Preheat the oven to 350°F (177°C). Place the pita pockets in the oven to warm, about 5 minutes.

Toss the seitan with the onion powder, garlic powder, cumin, paprika, thyme, salt, pepper and Worcestershire sauce.

In a large sauté pan, heat the extra-virgin olive oil until slick and shiny. Add the seitan to the sauté pan and sear on all sides until golden brown.

Spoon 1 teaspoon (3 g) of mayonnaise onto each pita pocket. Add 2 leaves romaine lettuce each, 3 tomato slices each and 3 slices of onion each.

Place 2 seitan slices in each pita pocket. Sprinkle with the cilantro, if using. Serve with mustard.

NUTRITIONAL INFORMATION PER SERVING: Calories: 280, Total Fat: 6 g, Saturated Fat: 0.5 g, Total Carbohydrates: 15 g, Fiber: 2 g, Net Carbohydrates: 13 g, Sugar: 3 g, Protein: 44 g, Sodium: 180 mg

CAULIFLOWER AND LEEK SOUP

SERVINGS: 4

Soups are a great way to fill up without filling out. The high water content will make you feel full and satisfied before you're able to overeat. The mild nuttiness of the cauliflower complements the sweet onion flavor of the leeks. Additionally, the silkiness of the pureed cauliflower makes this soup creamy without adding all of the unhealthy fat. This cauliflower and leek soup is so full of flavor and texture, it's sure to leave your taste buds satisfied.

1 tbsp (15 ml) extra-virgin olive oil

3 leeks, white parts only, chopped

2 cloves garlic, sliced

12 oz (340 g) cauliflower florets (about 1 small cauliflower)

3 cups (710 ml) vegetable stock

1 tsp salt

¼ tsp ground white pepper

TOPPING

1 tsp (5 ml) extra-virgin olive oil, plus more for drizzling

1 leek, green top and outer leaves removed, sliced thinly

Pinch of salt

Pinch of cayenne pepper

Pinch of dried parsley

In a medium stockpot, heat the extra-virgin olive oil over medium heat until slick and shiny. Add the leeks and garlic, and sauté for 2 to 3 minutes.

Add the cauliflower florets and sauté for another 4 to 5 minutes.

Add the vegetable stock, salt and white pepper. Bring to a light boil. Lower the heat to medium-low and let simmer for 20 to 25 minutes, or until the florets are completely soft and easily smashed by a fork.

Strain the soup and the leek mixture (separately reserving its liquid) into a blender. Blend until completely smooth. Add the reserved liquid (about ¾ cup [177 ml]) to the puree until the soup reaches your desired thickness.

For the topping: In a small sauté pan, heat the extra-virgin olive oil over high heat until slick and shiny. Add the leek and the salt, cayenne and parsley. Sauté for 2 to 3 minutes, until lightly browned at the edges and crispy.

Pour the soup into bowls and top with a sprinkle of crispy leek and a drizzle of extra-virgin olive oil.

NUTRITIONAL INFORMATION PER SERVING: Calories: 140, Total Fat: 6 g, Saturated Fat: 0.5 g, Total Carbohydrates: 21 g, Fiber: 4 g, Net Carbohydrates: 17 g, Sugar: 7 g, Protein: 4 g, Sodium: 795 mg

CALI BEAN BURGER

SERVINGS: MAKES ABOUT 10 PATTIES

Whether you're looking for something to impress your guests at your next BBQ or simply something to satisfy your burger craving, this recipe is your answer. The subtle earthiness of the black beans complements the more robust flavor of the kidney beans, creating the perfect blend. Additionally, the almond meal and flaxseeds add a nutty, meat-like flavor. The zesty smokiness of the chipotle lime aioli will send this recipe right to the top of your "favorites" list. While the ingredient list looks long, you can make these ahead of time and freeze for another time.

1 tsp (5 ml) extra-virgin olive oil

1 small onion, sliced

½ tsp balsamic vinegar

2 tsp (13 g) salt plus a pinch

1 (15 oz [425 g]) can red kidney beans, drained and rinsed

1 red bell pepper, coarsley chopped

2 cloves garlic, sliced

2 oz (57 g) kale, coarsley chopped

2 oz (57 g) canned or cooked black beans

¼ cup (34 g) whole wheat bread crumbs

2 tbsp (17 g) flaxseed meal + 2 tbsp (30 ml) water, mixed well

½ cup (48 g) almond meal

Pinch of cayenne pepper

Pinch of ground coriander

¼ tsp Old Bay seasoning

Pinch of ground cumin

¼ tsp black pepper

CHIPOTLE LIME AIOLI

Adobo sauce drained from 1 (4 oz [113 g]) can chipotle chiles

3 tbsp (26 g) vegan mayonnaise

Juice of ½ lime

PER BURGER

1 large leaf romaine lettuce

3 slices Roma tomato

2 slices avocado

Sprinkle of scallion, green parts only, cut into strips

(continued)

CALI BEAN BURGER (CONTINUED)

Preheat the oven to 375°F (190°C). Line a sheet pan with parchment paper.

In a medium sauté pan, heat the extra-virgin olive oil over medium heat until slick and shiny. Add the onion along with the balsamic vinegar and a pinch of salt. Sauté the onion until translucent, 3 to 4 minutes.

Lower the heat to low and let caramelize, about 30 minutes.

In a food processor, combine the caramelized onion, kidney beans, bell pepper, garlic, kale, black beans, bread crumbs, flaxseed mixture, almond meal, 2 teaspoons (10 g) of salt, and the cayenne, coriander, Old Bay, cumin and black pepper. Puree until a sticky dough forms.

Plastic wrap a mason jar lid and spray with nonstick spray. Scoop dough into the jar lid and smooth until level. Invert the jar lid to slide the patty onto the prepared sheet pan. Repeat to form the other burgers.

Bake the burgers for 20 to 25 minutes, until the outside is dry but the inside is lightly soft to the touch. Alternatively, cook over medium heat in a large sauté pan with a drizzle of the extra-virgin olive oil, about 5 minutes per side.

Let the burgers cool for 2 minutes.

Make the aioli: Whisk together the adobo sauce, mayonnaise and lime juice in small bowl until thoroughly combined.

To assemble each burger: Lay a romaine leaf on a plate. Add the tomatoes and avocado slices. Place the burger on top and spoon 1 teaspoon (3 g) of aioli on top. Garnish with the scallion.

NUTRITIONAL INFORMATION PER SERVING:
BURGER: Calories: 100, Total Fat: 4.5 g, Saturated Fat: 0 g, Total Carbohydrates: 11 g, Fiber: 4 g, Net Carbohydrates: 7 g, Sugar: 2 g, Protein: 5 g, Sodium: 550 mg
AIOLI: Calories: 15, Total Fat: 1 g, Saturated Fat: 0 g, Total Carbohydrates: 1 g, Fiber: 0 g, Net Carbohydrates: 1 g, Sugar: 0 g, Protein: 0 g, Sodium: 330 mg

SPICY TEMPEH SALAD

SERVINGS: 2

Tempeh is a fermented soy product that boasts an array of health benefits. Like many fermented foods, it is high in probiotics, or good bacteria, that help boost your immune system, fight off bad bacteria and aid in digestion. Additionally, tempeh's fermentation process leaves the isoflavones, which are naturally found in soy products, intact. These isoflavones are thought to help prevent bone loss, cardiovascular disease and some cancers. So grab a fork and dig into this delicious and nutritious spicy tempeh salad.

MARINATED TEMPEH

1 (8 oz [227 g]) package tempeh, diced

2 tbsp (30 ml) soy sauce

Pinch of cayenne pepper

1 clove garlic, sliced

1 scallion, sliced

1 tsp (5 g) dried oregano

Juice of 1 lime

1 tbsp (15 ml) + 1 tsp (5 ml) extra-virgin olive oil

DRESSING

1 tbsp (15 ml) extra-virgin olive oil

1 jalapeño chile, seeded and chopped

1 tsp (3 g) chopped fresh cilantro

Juice of ½ lime

Salt and black pepper

SALAD

4 oz (113 g) baby kale

2 oz (57 g) fennel, sliced thinly

½ avocado, diced

1 small red bell pepper, julienned

Make the tempeh: Combine the tempeh with all the marinade ingredients, except 1 tablespoon (15 ml) of the extra-virgin olive oil, and let sit overnight.

Strain the tempeh.

In a large sauté pan, heat the remaining 1 tablespoon (15 ml) of extra-virgin olive oil over medium-high heat. Sear the tempeh until golden brown on all sides.

Meanwhile, make the dressing: Puree all the dressing ingredients in a small blender, adding salt and black pepper to taste.

Combine the tempeh with the salad ingredients and toss with the dressing.

NUTRITIONAL INFORMATION PER SERVING:
MARINATED TEMPEH: Calories: 480, Total Fat: 32 g, Saturated Fat: 5 g, Total Carbohydrates: 29 g, Fiber: 7 g, Net Carbohydrates: 22 g, Sugar: 3 g, Protein: 27 g, Sodium: 2490 mg
DRESSING: Calories: 70, Total Fat: 7 g, Saturated Fat: 1 g, Total Carbohydrates: 0 g, Fiber: 0 g, Net Carbohydrates: 0 g, Sugar: 0 g, Protein: 0 g, Sodium: 80 mg

DINOSAUR KALE SALAD WITH ASIAN PEAR AND POMEGRANATE VINAIGRETTE

SERVINGS: 4 (AS AN APPETIZER)

Kale salads are great not only because they are super good for you, but also because they can be made a day in advance. The leaves are hearty enough that they won't wilt if you dress them ahead of time. This salad is filled to the brim with good nutrition—with vitamin K from the kale, omega-3 fatty acids from the walnuts and a plethora of antioxidants from the pomegranate. Besides being a nutritional powerhouse, it's beautiful, too, between the emerald green kale, garnet pomegranate seed gems and canary yellow Asian pear slices.

POMEGRANATE VINAIGRETTE

¼ cup (34 g) pomegranate arils

2 tbsp (30 ml) balsamic vinegar

2 tbsp (30 ml) extra-virgin olive oil

2 tsp (11 ml) Dijon mustard

½ tsp salt

1 tsp (3 g) black pepper

SALAD

¼ cup (34 g) chopped tempeh

6 cups (816 g) stemmed and chopped dinosaur (lacinato) kale

1 tsp (5 ml) extra-virgin olive oil

1 Asian pear, cored and sliced thinly

¼ cup (29 g) roughly chopped walnuts

¼ cup (34 g) pomegranate arils

Make the vinaigrette: In a small bowl, mash the pomegranate arils to make pomegranate juice.

Whisk together the rest of the dressing ingredients with the pomegranate juice, after you have discarded the pomegranate pulp. You can also put the ingredients in a small jar with a tight-fitting lid and shake well.

Make the salad: In a small sauté pan, cook the tempeh and heat over medium-high heat until browned on all sides.

Place the kale in a large bowl and drizzle with the extra-virgin olive oil. Massage the kale with your hands until you feel the greens soften.

Pour the dressing over the kale, tossing until the leaves are coated.

Top the salad with the tempeh, Asian pear and walnuts, then sprinkle with the pomegranate arils.

NUTRITIONAL INFORMATION PER SERVING:
SALAD: Calories: 150, Total Fat: 8 g, Saturated Fat: 1 g, Total Carbohydrates: 18 g, Fiber: 4 g, Net Carbohydrates: 14 g, Sugar: 4 g, Protein: 7 g, Sodium: 45 mg
DRESSING: Calories: 80, Total Fat: 7 g, Saturated Fat: 1 g, Total Carbohydrates: 4 g, Fiber: 1 g, Net Carbohydrates: 3 g, Sugar: 3 g, Protein: 0 g, Sodium: 350 mg

SUMMER GAZPACHO

SERVINGS: 4

Nothing tastes better on a warm evening than a nice, cool bowl of summer soup, and this gazpacho will definitely hit the spot. Plus, soups fill you up: Starting your meal with this yummy summer soup will keep you from overeating heavier main courses. So cool off and fill up with this delicious soup!

1 English (seedless) cucumber, chopped but not peeled

4 tomatoes, chopped, reserving 1 chopped tomato for garnish

1 red bell pepper, seeded and chopped

½ small red onion, chopped

½ stalk lemongrass, tough outer layer removed, stalk finely chopped

1 tbsp (9 g) minced fresh ginger

1½ tsp (4 g) garlic, minced

1 tbsp (15 ml) extra-virgin olive oil

2 tbsp (30 ml) red wine vinegar

2 tbsp (30 ml) fresh lemon juice

1½ cups (30 ml) low-sodium V8 juice

½ tsp (355 ml) sea salt

Black pepper

Dash of hot sauce and/or Worcestershire sauce (optional)

Place all the ingredients, except the reserved tomato and hot sauce, in a blender (not a food processor) and blend well.

Adjust the seasoning to your liking.

Refrigerate before serving.

Serve in bowls, topped with the reserved chopped tomato and a dash of hot sauce, if desired.

NUTRITIONAL INFORMATION PER SERVING: Calories: 110, Total Fat: 4.5 g, Saturated Fat: 0.5 g, Total Carbohydrates: 15 g, Fiber: 3 g, Net Carbohydrates: 12 g, Sugar: 6 g, Protein: 2 g, Sodium: 140 mg

CHAPTER 9

DINNER

Dinnertime is one of the best times of the day. Most people are just getting home after a long day of work and are ready to relax with a wonderful and warm meal shared with family. Dinnertime has gone through many changes in this county in the last several decades. In the 1950s, Mom made the meal and it mainly consisted of meat, starch and sometimes vegetables. In the 1980s, food was packaged and microwaved; in the 1990s, dinner was picked up at a drive-through window; and now it is somewhere in between, as there is a big push for eating "healthy." You may still make home-cooked meals, but there is too much take-out, packaged meals and dining out.

These recipes will bring you to a new time—it is like old meets new. They have the same nostalgia of long ago when meals were made at home and shared with family, but with a modern flair. No one has time to spend hours in the kitchen, but that doesn't mean health and nutrition should be sacrificed. Now you can have both: scrumptious and healthy meals, prepared at home in a quick and easy way.

The Zucchini Spaghetti with Vegetable Marinara (page 117) is not only the perfect solution for people who want to eat low-carb, but it takes five minutes to make, and it is so tasty you won't believe it's good for you. Or the BSM version of Eggplant Parmesan (page 121). You can make this on a weekend for either a traditional meal for a Sunday dinner with family, or have a dinner party and invite some friends over. They will be so thrilled to have a great-tasting meal that is also good for their waistline. For a Mexican-themed night, make the Black Bean and Roasted Vegetable Quesadilla with Spicy Pico de Gallo (page 126) and say olé!

ZUCCHINI SPAGHETTI WITH VEGETABLE MARINARA

SERVINGS: 2

One of my favorite things about spaghetti is its shape and texture. Now, thanks to vegetable spiralizing tools, you can get that same shape and texture without all of the unwanted blood sugar–spiking carbohydrates. Zucchini ribbons can be eaten raw or blanched for a slightly softer texture and are the perfect way to enjoy a childhood favorite—spaghetti with marinara sauce—in a healthful way.

1 tbsp (15 ml) extra-virgin olive oil

1 yellow onion, diced

⅛ tsp salt

8 oz (227 g) cremini mushrooms, sliced

1 tbsp (9 g) minced garlic

2 tbsp (30 ml) dry white wine

3 cups (408 g) heirloom tomatoes, chopped

2 cups (473 ml) vegetable stock

1 tbsp (9 g) herbes de Provence

Dash of sherry vinegar

Salt and black pepper

1 large zucchini, shredded or peeled with peeler into ribbons (use a spiralizer; e.g., Vegetti)

In a large rondeau or saucepot, heat the extra-virgin olive oil over medium heat until shiny. Add the onion and the salt. Sauté for 2 to 3 minutes.

Add the mushrooms and garlic and sauté for another 2 to 3 minutes.

Deglaze the pan with the white wine (it will sizzle) and let cook for 1 minute.

Add the tomatoes, stock and herbs. Bring the mixture to a boil and then lower the heat to medium-low.

Cook, uncovered, for 1 hour. Roughly halfway through, add the sherry vinegar. The mixture should resemble a vegetable stew by the end—roughly half of the liquid should be evaporated.

Puree in a blender to the desired coarseness, adding salt and pepper to taste.

Return the mixture to the pot and add the zucchini. Cook for 1 to 2 minutes.

NUTRITIONAL INFORMATION PER SERVING:
PASTA: Calories: 25 g, Total Fat: 0.5 g, Saturated Fat: 0 g, Total Carbohydrates: 5 g, Fiber: 1 g, Net Carbohydrates: 4 g, Sugar: 3 g, Protein: 2 g, Sodium: 15 mg
VEGETABLE MARINARA SAUCE: Calories: 60, Total Fat: 2 g, Saturated Fat: 0 g, Total Carbohydrates: 6 g, Fiber: 1 g, Net Carbohydrates: 5 g, Sugar: 1 g, Protein: 2 g, Sodium: 320 mg

LOUISIANA RED BEANS AND SMOKED TEMPEH WITH QUINOA AND SWISS CHARD SAUTÉ

SERVINGS: 2

This dish is a take on traditional red beans and rice with tons of extra nutrition and satisfying protein. Choosing smoked tempeh adds a robust, meaty flavor while skipping the saturated fat. High in fiber, protein and B vitamins, quinoa is an ancient grain that adds soft texture to the dish. The flowing Swiss chard ribbons not only add bulk with few calories, but the vibrant colors complement the red beans beautifully.

SMOKED TEMPEH

2 tbsp (30 ml) extra-virgin olive oil

4 oz (113 g) yellow onion, minced

2 cloves garlic, minced

1 green bell pepper, minced

1 rib celery, minced

1 oz (30 ml) red wine

1 (15 oz [425 g]) can red kidney beans, drained and rinsed

Pinch of cayenne pepper

¼ tsp dried thyme

1 dash dried sage

¼ tsp dried parsley

1 tsp (2 g) Cajun seasoning

Salt and black pepper

½ cup (118 ml) vegetable stock

8 oz (227 g) smoked tempeh or tofu, sliced into strips

QUINOA AND CHARD

1 cup (237 ml) water

½ cup (68 g) uncooked quinoa

1 tbsp (15 ml) extra-virgin olive oil

1 bunch red chard, stemmed and chopped

1 clove garlic, minced

Salt and black pepper

Prepare the smoked tempeh: Heat the extra-virgin olive oil in a large sauté pan until slick and shiny.

Add the onion, garlic, bell pepper and celery and cook for 3 to 4 minutes, until the onion is translucent. Deglaze with the red wine.

Add the kidney beans and all the seasonings, including salt and black pepper to taste. Sauté for 1 to 2 minutes.

Add the vegetable stock and smoked tempeh and stir. Cover and simmer until most of the stock is absorbed and the tofu is heated through.

Prepare the quinoa and chard: In a medium stockpot, heat the water and quinoa over medium-high heat. When the water reaches a boil, lower the heat to low and cover. Cook until the water is absorbed and the quinoa is cooked, about 10 minutes.

Heat the extra-virgin olive oil in a sauté pan until slick and shiny. Add the chard along with the garlic, and salt and black pepper to taste. Sauté for 2 to 3 minutes. Add the quinoa and sauté for another 30 seconds. Serve the tempeh with the quinoa and chard.

NUTRITIONAL INFORMATION PER SERVING: Calories: 788, Total Fat: 37 g, Saturated Fat: 5 g, Total Carbohydrates: 79 g, Fiber: 14 g, Net Carbohydrates: 64 g, Sugar: 10 g, Protein: 40 g, Sodium: 926 mg

OUTRAGEOUSLY GOOD HOMEMADE VEGGIE BURGERS

SERVINGS: 6

Store-bought veggie burgers can be laden with sodium, calories and preservatives. These homemade burgers are packed with flavor, whole foods and nutrition. Choosing lentils as the base for the dish provides the body with essential protein, carbohydrates, fiber and magnesium. Not only will this keep you fuller longer, but magnesium plays a key role in digestion.

Extra-virgin olive oil spray

2 tbsp (30 ml) coconut oil

2 shallots, chopped small

1 rib celery, chopped small

1 large carrot, grated

1 cup (136 g) cremini mushrooms, chopped small

2 cloves garlic, minced

1 (15 oz [425 g]) can lentils, drained and rinsed

½ tsp salt

¼ tsp black pepper

½ tsp paprika

¾ cup (102 g) whole wheat bread crumbs

1 tsp (5 ml) soy sauce

1 tbsp (9 g) finely chopped fresh cilantro

1 tbsp (9 g) flaxseed meal + 3 tbsp (45 ml) water, mixed well

2 ripe avocados, divided into thirds and sliced

1 medium tomato, sliced

Romaine lettuce

Preheat the oven to 350°F (177°C) . Line a cookie sheet with aluminum foil and spray lightly with extra-virgin olive oil spray.

In a nonstick pan, heat 1 tablespoon (15 ml) of the coconut oil and sauté the shallots, celery, carrot, mushrooms and garlic for about 5 minutes, until the vegetables are softened.

Set the cooked vegetables aside to cool.

In a food processor, puree the lentils and then transfer to a large bowl. Next, pulse the vegetables in the food processor until mostly smooth, with some small chunks. Add this to the pureed lentils.

To the lentil mixture, add the salt, pepper, paprika, bread crumbs, soy sauce, cilantro and flaxseed mixture. Combine until all the ingredients are incorporated.

Form the mixture into 6 patties, each about ½-inch (13-cm) thick.

Using a paper towel, wipe out the nonstick pan used before and heat ½ tablespoon (7 ml) of the coconut oil over medium-high heat. Place 3 burgers in the pan and cook on each side for 2 to 3 minutes, until lightly browned. Remove from the pan and set aside.

Place the remaining ½ tablespoon (7 ml) of coconut oil in the pan and cook the last 3 burgers.

Place the burgers on the prepared cookie sheet and cook in the oven for 20 minutes.

Serve warm with slices of avocado, tomato and lettuce.

NUTRITIONAL INFORMATION PER SERVING: Calories: 284, Total Fat: 14 g, Saturated Fat: 5 g, Total Carbohydrates: 33 g, Fiber: 12 g, Net Carbohydrates: 21 g, Sugar: 5 g, Protein: 10 g, Sodium: 363 mg

SPICY CHANA MASALA

SERVINGS: 4

This spice-filled dish boasts flavors and ingredients from around the globe. The spice blend will not only awaken your taste buds, but such spices as cinnamon, fennel and fenugreek have been shown to help with blood sugar control. Red chili flakes will add a nice heat to the dish while providing capsaicin, a phytochemical that may help increase metabolism.

MASALA

1 oz (28 g) dried coconut pieces

1 cinnamon stick

1 tsp (3 g) fennel seeds

¼ tsp mustard seeds

1½ tsp (4 g) cumin seeds

1 tsp (3 g) coriander seeds

½ tsp fenugreek

¼ tsp red chili flakes

2 cloves

½ cup (118 ml) water

2 tbsp (30 ml) extra-virgin olive oil

6 oz (170 g) yellow onion, diced

12 curry leaves

½ tsp ground turmeric

1 tsp (3 g) minced garlic

1 tsp (5 g) minced fresh ginger

1 tsp (2 g) paprika

2 Roma tomatoes, diced

2 (15 oz [425 g]) cans garbanzo beans (chickpeas), drained and rinsed

2 tsp (10 ml) soy sauce

1 tbsp (9 g) chopped fresh cilantro

Make the masala: In a sauté pan, toast the coconut, cinnamon, fennel, mustard, cumin and coriander seeds, fenugeek, red chili flakes and cloves over medium heat for 3 to 4 minutes, until the coconut is golden brown. Remove from the heat and let cool.

Puree the mixture with the water and set aside.

Heat the extra-virgin olive oil in a medium sauté pan over medium heat until the oil is slick and shiny. Add the onion. Sauté for 2 to 3 minutes, until the onion is translucent.

Add the curry leaves, turmeric, garlic, ginger and paprika and sauté for 1 minute. Add the tomatoes and sauté for 1 minute. Add the masala and sauté for 1 minute.

Add the garbanzo beans and soy sauce. Sauté until the masala has a drier, paste-like consistency and shows toasty brown edges.

Serve with the cilantro.

NUTRITIONAL INFORMATION PER SERVING: Calories: 374, Total Fat: 14 g, Saturated Fat: 5 g, Total Carbohydrates: 46 g, Fiber: 12 g, Net Carbohydrates: 34 g, Total Sugar: 3 g, Protein: 14 g, Sodium: 582 mg

SKINNY EGGPLANT PARMESAN

SERVINGS: 4

This recipe takes a classic comfort food and turns it into cute individual portions that are not only tasty, but much healthier than the original. This recipe has all of the taste but none of the guilt. It is significantly lower in fat and calories than the traditional version. Serve with a side green salad and maybe even some sautéed spinach for an extra dose of greens.

VEGAN PARMESAN

½ cup (56 g) raw cashews

2 tbsp (19 g) nutritional yeast

½ tsp salt

Pinch of garlic powder

1 large eggplant, unpeeled, sliced into thick rounds

Salt

1 tsp (3 g) cornstarch

½ cup (118 ml) unsweetened soy milk

1 cup (121 g) panko bread crumbs

2 tbsp (23 g) vegan Parmesan cheese

¼ tsp dried rosemary

¼ tsp dried thyme

¼ tsp dried oregano

Pinch of black pepper

¼ cup (31 g) all-purpose flour

Extra-virgin olive oil

Preheat the oven to 400°F (204°C).

To make the vegan Parmesan, combine the cashews, yeast, salt and garlic powder and process in a food processor.

Salt the eggplant slices liberally and set on paper towels for 10 minutes. Rinse the eggplant and dry with paper towels.

Combine the cornstarch with the soy milk in one bowl.

Combine the bread crumbs, vegan Parmesan, rosemary, thyme, oregano, ¼ teaspoon of salt and the black pepper in another bowl.

Dip the eggplant into the flour to coat, then into the soy milk mixture, then into the bread crumb mixture. Arrange on a baking sheet and bake for 20 minutes.

Heat the extra-virgin olive oil in a large sauté pan until slick and shiny.

Panfry the eggplant slices for 2 minutes on each side to make them extra crispy.

Serve with Zucchini Spaghetti with Vegetable Marinara (page 117).

NUTRITIONAL INFORMATION PER ROUND: Calories: 51, Total Fat: 3 g, Saturated Fat: 0.4 g, Total Carbohydrates: 6.6 g, Fiber: 1.2 g, Net Carbohydrates: 5.4 g, Sugar: 1.1 g, Protein: 0.5 g, Sodium: 130 mg

VEGETABLE LASAGNE WITH CASHEW RICOTTA

SERVINGS: 4

Zucchini has become increasingly popular as a replacement for pasta noodles, as their light flavor makes them versatile, and because zucchini tastes amazing when paired with tomato sauces. This vegan version is much lighter and more refreshing than its counterpart, but its flavor packs just as much punch! Serve it with an arugula salad for a meal that will leave you fully satisfied.

1 tbsp (15 ml) extra-virgin olive oil

1 medium onion, diced

1 (8 oz [227 g]) package ground seitan

2 portobello mushrooms, diced

Zucchini: middle sections left over from making the Pistou (page 103), diced

2 cloves garlic, minced

2 sprigs rosemary, leaves only, chopped

1 sprig thyme, leaves only

1 tbsp (15 ml) white wine

2 cups (322 g) diced San Marzano tomatoes

Salt and black pepper

Pinch of red chili pepper (optional)

1 cup (230 g) Cashew Dream Cheese (page 171)

½ cup (20 g) fresh basil, chopped

3 zucchini, sliced with vegetable peeler

Preheat the oven to 375°F (190°C).

In a large sauté pan, heat the extra-virgin olive oil over medium heat until slick and shiny. Add the onion, seitan, mushrooms, zucchini pieces, garlic, rosemary and thyme. Sauté for 4 to 5 minutes, until the onion is translucent.

Add the white wine. Sauté for 1 minute. Add the tomatoes and season to taste with salt, black pepper and red chili pepper, if using. Simmer for 10 minutes on low heat. Remove from the heat and let cool.

Stir in the Cashew Dream Cheese and basil.

Coat the bottom of a casserole pan with the zucchini slices, overlapping slightly. Spoon an even layer of filling over the zucchini. Add another layer of zucchini slices, overlapping slightly. Spoon another even layer of filling over the zucchini. Continue until all the filling is used, ending with a layer of zucchini slices on top.

Bake for 15 to 20 minutes, or until the filling is bubbling at the edges.

Let cool for 5 minutes before slicing.

NUTRITIONAL INFORMATION PER SERVING: Calories: 265, Total Fat: 11.6 g, Saturated Fat: 1.8 g, Total Carbohydrates: 28.4 g, Fiber: 5.1 g, Net Carbohydrates: 23.3 g, Sugar: 6.8 g, Protein: 13.9 g, Sodium: 509 mg

QUINOA-STUFFED BELL PEPPERS

SERVINGS: 4

These savory stuffed peppers make the perfect lunch, dinner or side dish. Choosing quinoa, tempeh and mushrooms as the base for the stuffing provides this dish with plenty of plant-based protein and meaty flavor. Feel free to get creative and add any vegetables you have on hand; carrots, zucchini and eggplant would all be wonderful additions.

¼ cup (53 g) uncooked quinoa

½ cup (118 ml) water

¼ cup (32 g) chopped leek

½ cup (38 g) cremini mushrooms, stemmed and chopped

4 oz (113 g) tempeh, chopped

1 tbsp (9 g) sun-dried tomatoes, chopped

1 clove garlic, minced

Pinch of salt

Pinch of black pepper

1 tbsp (15 ml) white wine

2 tbsp (30 ml) vegetable stock

2 red bell peppers, halved and cored

Preheat the oven to 350°F (177°C).

Place the quinoa and water in a small stockpot. Bring to a boil. Lower the heat, cover and simmer for about 10 minutes. Once the water evaporates, remove from the heat.

In a medium sauté pan over medium heat, combine the leek, mushrooms, tempeh, tomatoes, garlic, salt and black pepper. Sauté for 3 to 5 minutes, or until the leek is soft.

Deglaze with the wine. Add the vegetable stock and let simmer for 5 minutes.

Remove the pan from the heat and add the quinoa. Stir to mix thoroughly.

Scoop the mixture into the bell pepper halves. Bake for 5 minutes.

Remove from the oven and let cool for 5 minutes.

NUTRITIONAL INFORMATION PER SERVING: Calories: 126, Total Fat: 4 g, Saturated Fat: 1 g, Total Carbohydrates: 15 g, Fiber: 2 g, Net Carbohydrates: 13 g, Sugar: 3 g, Protein: 8 g, Sodium: 102 mg

ROASTED PORTOBELLO BURGER

SERVINGS: 2

Grilled portobello caps have a body to them that is reminiscent of a burger, but don't leave you feeling weighed down or tired. Instead of French fries, try pairing these burgers with root vegetable sticks, a green salad or any veggie side dish.

CARAMELIZED ONIONS

1 tsp (5 ml) extra-virgin olive oil

1 medium yellow onion, sliced

Salt and black pepper

3 cloves garlic, minced

1 cup (136 g) chopped dinosaur kale

¼ cup (59 ml) + 1 tbsp (15 ml) vegetable stock

2 portobello mushrooms, left whole

PER BURGER

2 slices sprouted-grain bread (e.g., Ezekiel brand)

1 tsp (5 g) vegan mayonnaise

1 thick slice tomato

2 leaves romaine lettuce

Make the caramelized onions: Heat the extra-virgin olive oil over medium heat in a large skillet. Add the onion slices and cook, stirring often, for 25 minutes, until the onion is cooked through, translucent and caramelized. Season with salt and pepper to taste. Remove from the pan and set aside.

In the same pan, heat the garlic over medium heat. Add the kale and the 1 tablespoon (15 ml) of vegetable stock and cook for 3 to 4 minutes, until the kale is wilted. Remove from the heat and set aside.

Heat a separate large skillet or grill pan over high heat. Place the portobello mushrooms and the remaining ¼ cup (59 ml) of vegetable stock in the pan and cook for 3 to 4 minutes per side.

Assemble each burger: On a slice of bread, layer a portobello and the mayonnaise, tomato slice, romaine, half of the kale and half of the caramelized onions, then top with the second slice of bread.

NUTRITIONAL INFORMATION PER SERVING: Calories: 261, Total Fat: 12.2 g, Saturated Fat: 0.7 g, Total Carbohydrates: 29.4 g, Fiber: 18.3 g, Net Carbohydrates: 11.1 g, Sugar: 4.6 g, Protein: 17.8 g, Sodium: 381 mg

MISO-MARINATED TOFU WITH SESAME BROCCOLI

SERVINGS: 2

Tofu is a wonderful ingredient to cook with because it's so versatile; it takes on the flavors of whatever sauce you put it in. It's also high in protein, which helps maintain blood sugar levels and satiety throughout the day. This wonderful miso soy marinade is great; it's so flavorful that even with a short marinating time, the tofu will soak up all of the flavor.

2 tsp (6 g) white miso

2 tsp (10 ml) soy sauce

1 tbsp (3 g) fresh cilantro, chopped

1 clove garlic, sliced

2 tbsp (6 g) scallion, chopped

1 tbsp (14 g) fresh ginger, sliced

1 tsp (5 ml) sesame oil

1 tsp (5 ml) mirin

¼ cup (60 ml) water

8 oz (227 g) tofu, sliced into thin rectangles

4 oz (113 g) Chinese broccoli or broccolini, stems trimmed

2 tsp (10 ml) sesame oil

2 oz (56 g) yellow onion, sliced

1 tsp (5 ml) soy sauce

Sprinkle of black or white sesame seeds

Combine the miso, soy sauce, cilantro, garlic, scallion, ginger, sesame oil, mirin and water in a large bowl and whisk to incorporate.

Add the tofu and let marinate for 30 minutes.

Bring a medium stockpot three-quarters full of salted water to a rolling boil. Add the broccoli to the pot and blanch for 1 minute. Shock immediately in ice water and spin dry.

In a medium sauté pan, heat the sesame oil over medium heat until slick and shiny.

Add the onion and sauté for 2 to 3 minutes, until the onion is translucent.

Add the broccoli and soy sauce. Sauté for 1 to 2 minutes, until the broccoli is heated through.

Remove from the heat and sprinkle with sesame seeds.

Serve with the marinated tofu.

NUTRITIONAL INFORMATION PER SERVING:
DRESSING: Calories: 160, Total Fat: 8 g, Saturated Fat: 1 g, Total Carbohydrates: 8 g, Fiber: 2 g, Net Carbohydrates: 6 g, Sugar: 2 g, Protein: 13 g, Sodium: 460 mg
DISH: Calories: 160, Total Fat: 11 g, Saturated Fat: 1.5 g, Total Carbohydrates: 15 g, Fiber: 4 g, Net Carbohydrates: 11 g, Sugar: 2 g, Protein: 4 g, Sodium: 85 mg

BLACK BEAN AND ROASTED VEGETABLE QUESADILLA WITH SPICY PICO DE GALLO

SERVINGS: 4

Nutritional yeast is an incredible addition to any kitchen. Not only does it give you that cheesy taste without the unwanted saturated fat, it also provides a whole host of nutritional benefits. For one, it's the only vegetarian source of vitamin B_{12}, essential for proper metabolism. On top of that, it contains all eighteen essential amino acids! Sprinkle it on top of mashed avocado and black beans for the tastiest—and healthiest—quesadilla you've ever tried.

QUESADILLA

½ avocado, mashed

1 (10″ [25.4 cm]) sprouted whole-grain tortilla (e.g., Ezekiel brand)

Salt and black pepper

2 tsp (6 g) nutritional yeast

2 oz (57 g) canned or cooked black beans

4 oz (113 g) roasted red pepper, diced

½ oz (14 g) red onion, mandolined or sliced thinly

Pinch of ground cumin

Pinch of paprika

PICO DE GALLO

1 oz (28 g) red onion, cut into small dice

3 oz (85 g) tomato, seeded and cut into small dice

1 serrano chile (2 for extra spicy), seeded and cut into small dice

1 tbsp (3 g) chopped fresh cilantro

Juice of ¼ lime

Salt and black pepper

Make the quesadilla: Spread the mashed avocado on half of the tortilla and sprinkle with a pinch each of salt and pepper. Sprinkle the nutritional yeast on top.

Layer on the black beans and roasted red pepper. Spread the red onion in one even layer.

Add the cumin and paprika on top with another pinch each of salt and pepper.

Fold the quesadilla over onto itself and press down lightly.

Heat a large sauté pan or grill pan over high heat for 2 to 3 minutes. Place the quesadilla in the pan and grill for 2 minutes on each side.

Remove from the pan and cut into 4 pieces.

Make the pico de gallo: Combine all the ingredients in small bowl. Season with salt and pepper to taste. Mix to incorporate.

Serve with the quesadilla.

NUTRITIONAL INFORMATION PER SERVING:
QUESADILLA: Calories: 220, Total Fat: 18.5 g, Saturated Fat: 1 g, Total Carbohydrates: 31 g, Fiber: 9 g, Net Carbohydrates: 22 g, Sugar: 1 g, Protein: 8 g, Sodium: 280 mg
PICO DE GALLO: Calories: 10, Total Fat: 0 g, Saturated Fat: 0 g, Total Carbohydrates: 2 g, Fiber: 0 g, Net Carbohydrates: 2 g, Sugar: 1 g, Protein: 0 g, Sodium: 40 mg

HARISSA-SPICED WHITE BEAN AND VEGETABLE "MASH" (VEGAN SHEPHERD'S PIE)

SERVINGS: 3

Shepherd's pie was a favorite for so many of us while we were growing up, and it's often still thought of as a comfort food. Luckily, you can indulge in this delicious vegan version guilt-free. It's chock-full of phytonutrients from the variety of vegetables and has plenty of satiating protein from the seitan, but still has the hearty taste of the original. And making it is easy as pie.

2 tbsp (30 ml) extra-virgin olive oil

4 oz (113 g) ground seitan

4 oz (113 g) diced yellow onion

2 cloves garlic, minced

2 oz (57 g) diced celery

2 oz (57 g) diced carrots

4 oz (113 g) stemmed and diced shiitake mushrooms

2 sprigs thyme, leaves only

1 tbsp (15 ml) red wine

1 cup (237 ml) vegetable stock

Salt and black pepper

1 (15 oz [425 g]) can cannellini beans, drained and rinsed

1 tbsp (16 g) harissa

1 tbsp (3 g) chopped fresh parsley

In a large sauté pan, heat 1 tablespoon (15 ml) of the extra-virgin olive oil over medium heat until slick and shiny.

Add the seitan, onion, garlic, celery, carrots, shiitake mushrooms and thyme. Sauté for 4 to 5 minutes until the onion is translucent and the shiitakes have reduced in size by half.

Add the red wine and sauté for 1 minute.

Add ½ cup (118 ml) of the vegetable stock and sauté for another 10 minutes, until the carrots are crisp but cooked through. Season with salt and black pepper.

In a small pot, combine the cannellini beans with the remaining ½ cup (118 ml) of vegetable stock, harissa, ½ teaspoon of salt and ¼ teaspoon of pepper. Bring to a soft boil and let cook until all the liquid is absorbed.

Puree the bean mixture with the parsley and up to 1 tablespoon (15 ml) of the remaining extra-virgin olive oil to the desired level of smoothness.

Serve in bowls with the seitan mixture at the bottom, covered with a layer of the bean mixture à la classic shepherd's pie.

NUTRITIONAL INFORMATION PER SERVING: Calories: 390, Total Fat: 12 g, Saturated Fat: 1.5 g, Total Carbohydrates: 35 g, Fiber: 9 g, Net Carbohydrates: 26 g, Sugar: 6 g, Protein: 37 g, Sodium: 675 mg

ONE-POT VEGETARIAN SAUTÉ

SERVINGS: 4

Looking for a gourmet-tasting meal with almost no cleanup? So was I, which is why I developed this exquisite one-pot vegetarian sauté. A combination of hearty protein from the beans and vegetarian sausage links, healthy fats from the pine nuts and healthy carbohydrates from the vegetables make this meal perfectly balanced. Balanced, easy to make and little cleanup? This dish is a no-brainer!

1 tbsp (15 ml) extra-virgin olive oil

2 cloves garlic, chopped

10 Brussels sprouts, sliced thinly

6 oz (170 g) vegetarian sausage links

½ tsp dried thyme

½ (15 oz [213 g]) can cannellini beans, drained and rinsed

1 tsp (3 g) black pepper

Dash of white wine

1 (15 oz [425 g]) jar roasted red peppers, sliced

½ cup (75 g) pea pods

1 tbsp (8 g) pine nuts

In a medium sauté pan, combine the extra-virgin olive oil and garlic. Sauté for 1 minute over medium heat.

Add all the remaining ingredients, except the pine nuts, to the pan and cook until the vegetables are tender yet crisp. Sprinkle with pine nuts to taste.

NUTRITIONAL INFORMATION PER SERVING: Calories: 300, Total Fat: 4 g, Saturated Fat: 0.5 g, Total Carbohydrates: 42 g, Fiber: 7 g, Net Carbohydrates: 35 g, Sugar 8 g, Protein: 19 g, Sodium: 301 mg

GINGER-LEMONGRASS STIR-FRY

SERVINGS: 2

This fun stir-fry will make your kitchen smell incredible! The zingy flavor of the lemongrass is so completely unique and isn't commonly found in American dishes, so this dish introduces something new and very special! It is easy to make and can last for days, so feel free to double up on the recipe to have leftovers for the next day.

3 tbsp (45 ml) extra-virgin olive oil

2 stalks lemongrass

5 oz (142 g) extra-firm tofu, cubed

1 red bell pepper, julienned

1 oz (28 g) red onion, sliced

4 oz (113 g) snow peas, trimmed

2 oz (57 g) bamboo shoots, drained

1 tsp (5 g) minced fresh ginger

2 tsp (10 g) soy sauce

In a wok or large sauté pan, heat the extra-virgin olive oil over high heat until slick and shiny.

Add the lemongrass stalks and sauté for 4 to 5 minutes, until highly fragrant.

Remove the lemongrass from the wok and discard. Lower the heat to medium.

Add the tofu, bell pepper, onion, snow peas, bamboo shoots, ginger and soy sauce.

Sauté for 4 to 5 minutes, until the onion is translucent, the snow peas are bright green and the tofu is lightly browned.

NUTRITIONAL INFORMATION PER SERVING: Calories: 369, Total Fat: 24.7 g, Saturated Fat: 1.6 g, Total Carbohydrates: 30.7 g, Fiber: 4.8 g, Net Carbohydrates: 25.9 g, Sugar: 6.7 g, Protein: 11.1 g, Sodium: 322 mg

CHAPTER 10

SIDES, SNACKS AND TREATS

It is really difficult to find healthy snacks on the go today. Stores and airports are lined with candy bars, chips and over-the-top sugary snacks. What is one to do? With just a little planning, you can have healthy and great-tasting snacks. Snacking doesn't have to be unhealthy. It can be a part of nutritious diet. First, it's important not to go too long without eating—if you wait too long and get too hungry, you will be more inclined to overeat at your next meal, or you will make a poor choice because you are starving. Second, properly planned snacks will help keep your blood sugar stable during the day. Third, healthy snacking can be a great way to get in a serving of fruits and veggies!

The BSM Crunchy Chickpeas (page 147) are a great way to satisfy your need to "crunch" while providing a dose of fiber and nutrients. They can be made ahead of time and thrown into your bag to take to work. They are also a great snack to pack while traveling. For an extra treat and to satisfy your sweet craving, try our Antioxidant Chocolate Coins (page 145) or our Homemade Strawberry Ice Cream (page 141).

ZA'ATAR FLAXSEED HUMMUS

SERVINGS: 4

This hummus is far less complicated than the number of ingredients suggests. Not only is the preparation incredibly simple, but this hummus will last for several days in the fridge once complete. If you make enough at one time for a few days' supply, then you can combine this recipe with some veggie sticks for a grab-and-go snack!

1 cup (201 g) uncooked red lentils

1 cup (237 ml) cold water

1 tbsp (9 g) za'atar

1 tsp (5 g) salt

¼ tsp ground black pepper

2 oz (62 ml) extra-virgin olive oil

1 tbsp (3 g) fresh cilantro, chopped

1 clove garlic, sliced

1 tbsp (9 g) ground flaxseeds

Juice of ¼ lemon

1 tbsp (3 g) chives, chopped

Combine the lentils and water in small stockpot and bring to a light boil. Lower the heat to low. Simmer, uncovered, for 30 to 40 minutes, until the lentils are completely cooked and absorb all the liquid. The lentils should have a creamy consistency. Remove from the heat and let cool.

Combine the lentils, za'atar, salt, black pepper, extra-virgin olive oil, cilantro, garlic, flaxseeds, lemon juice and chives in a food processor and process until very smooth.

NUTRITIONAL INFORMATION PER SERVING (2 tbsp): Calories: 202, Total Fat: 15.6 g, Saturated Fat: 2 g, Total Carbohydrates: 11.5 g, Fiber: 5 g, Net Carbohydrates: 6.5 g, Sugar: 1.1 g, Protein: 5.2 g, Sodium: 8 mg

EGGPLANT SPREAD

SERVINGS: 6

The deep purple color of eggplant is indicative of the nutrients this funny-shaped vegetable packs inside. Copper, vitamin B$_1$, magnesium, vitamin B$_6$ and phytonutrients are just a few. The texture of eggplant when cooked, very soft and a bit pulpy, is perfect for dips and spreads like this one. Enjoy this eggplant dip with some fresh veggies for an afternoon snack or as a filling dinner appetizer.

2 small to medium eggplants

1 tsp (1 g) fresh oregano, stemmed

1 tbsp (3 g) chopped fresh parsley

½ tsp chopped garlic

1 tsp (3 g) tahini

2 tbsp (30 ml) extra-virgin olive oil

2 tbsp (30 ml) lemon juice

Salt and black pepper

Preheat the oven to 450°F (232°C). Prick the eggplants with a fork and roast in a casserole dish until soft, 30 to 45 minutes.

Remove from the oven and let cool.

Scoop out the eggplant flesh and puree with the rest of the ingredients, seasoning with salt and black pepper to taste.

NUTRITIONAL INFORMATION PER SERVING: Calories: 90, Total Fat: 5 g, Saturated Fat: 1 g, Total Carbohydrates: 9 g, Fiber: 5 g, Net Carbohydrates: 4 g, Sugar: 4 g, Protein: 2 g, Sodium: 390 mg

SWEET POTATO FRIES

SERVINGS: 4

These fries are a great substitute for original French fries. For one, they are baked instead of fried, so that saves you a lot of fat and calories right there. And sweet potatoes are high in beta-carotene and fiber, which adds to their appeal. This recipe is so tasty and nutritious, you won't even miss the frying.

2 large sweet potatoes, peeled and cut into strips

2 tbsp (30 ml) extra-virgin olive oil

½ tsp chili powder

¼ tsp salt

Black pepper

Preheat the oven to 450°F (232°C). Line a baking sheet with aluminum foil.

Place the sweet potatoes in a large bowl and toss them with the extra-virgin olive oil until coated. Add the chili powder, salt and black pepper to taste and toss again.

Arrange the sweet potatoes in a single layer on the prepared pan. Bake for 20 minutes on the lower rack.

Transfer to the upper rack and bake for 10 more minutes, or until crispy.

NUTRITIONAL INFORMATION PER SERVING: Calories: 116, Total Fat: 7 g, Saturated Fat: 1 g, Total Carbohydrates: 13 g, Fiber: 2 g, Net Carbohydrates: 11 g, Sugar: 3 g, Protein: 1 g, Sodium: 196 mg

SPICY GUACAMOLE

SERVINGS: 6

With only four ingredients, it can't get much easier than this delicious guacamole. The acidity of the lemon juice balances out the creaminess of the avocados, and the picante sauce gives the dip a slight kick. Paired with some crunchy vegetables—my favorite is subtly sweet jicama—this dip makes for the perfect afternoon snack. The healthy fats from the avocados will help fill you up and keep you satisfied until dinner.

3 large avocados

3 tbsp (45 ml) lemon juice

3 tbsp (26 g) medium picante sauce

1 tsp (5 g) salt (optional)

Mash all the ingredients together and enjoy with vegetables. Try with jicama.

NUTRITIONAL INFORMATION PER SERVING: Calories: 160, Total Fat: 15 g, Saturated Fat: 2 g, Total Carbohydrates: 10 g, Fiber: 7 g, Net Carbohydrates: 3 g, Sugar: 1 g, Protein: 2 g, Sodium: 430 mg

CHICKPEA SPREAD

SERVINGS: 15

Smooth and creamy, this dip is perfect for dipping or spreading. It's delicious scooped onto crunchy veggies or dolloped onto a hearty salad, or even as a condiment on your favorite sandwich. You can't go wrong with this chickpea spread. And with its healthy dose of protein, fiber and magnesium—three nutrients that play a major role in good glucose control—you won't have to worry about your meal's or snack's effect on your blood sugar.

2 cups (402 g) canned or cooked garbanzo beans (chickpeas)

½ tsp salt

3 cloves garlic, chopped finely

½ cup (118 ml) vegetable oil

¼ cup (60 ml) lemon juice

2 tbsp (5 g) chopped fresh parsley (optional)

Drain and wash the chickpeas under cold water and place on a paper towel to dry.

Blend all the ingredients, at high speed, for 10 seconds.

Serve with fresh vegetables.

NUTRITIONAL INFORMATION PER SERVING: Calories: 100, Total Fat: 8 g, Saturated Fat: 1 g, Total Carbohydrates: 6 g, Fiber: 2 g, Net Carbohydrates: 4 g, Sugar: 0 g, Protein: 2 g, Sodium: 80 mg

PICO DE GALLO SALSA

SERVINGS: 2

This pico de gallo is more than just a salsa; it's a fresh and juicy salad that can be enjoyed on its own or as a side dish, a zesty topping for tacos and wraps and a tasty addition to delicious veggie scrambles. Bursting with flavor, extremely versatile and easy to make, it's the perfect recipe to make ahead of time and use on multiple dishes throughout the week.

2 Roma tomatoes

¼ cup (38 g) diced yellow onion

Juice of ½ lime

⅛ cup (21 g) diced jalapeño chile

A few sprigs of cilantro, chopped

¼ tsp salt

Black pepper

Mix all the ingredients together, including the black pepper to taste, and enjoy!

NUTRITIONAL INFORMATION PER SERVING: Calories: 25, Total Fat: 0 g, Saturated Fat: 0 g, Total Carbohydrates: 5 g, Fiber: 1 g, Net Carbohydrates: 4 g, Sugar: 2 g, Protein: 1 g, Sodium: 190 mg

SPICY POPCORN

SERVINGS: 2 CUPS (272 G)

I can't begin to explain how much I love popcorn! This low-calorie, whole-grain snack is loaded with fiber and antioxidants to help keep you fuller longer and prevent spikes in blood sugar between meals. Spicy snacks are a great way to rev up the metabolism, but feel free to spice up your kernels any way you choose. Some of my favorite combinations are fresh lemon zest and coarsely ground black pepper, garlic powder and aminos, or for a dessert option, try ground cinnamon and nutmeg with a pinch of ground cloves.

---

2 tbsp (30 ml) extra-virgin olive oil

½ cup (68 g) unpopped popcorn kernels

¼ cup (57 g) vegan butter

2 tbsp (30 ml) of your favorite hot sauce

1 tsp (5 g) salt

¼ tsp red chili flakes

Pinch of cayenne pepper

Juice of ½ lemon

In large sauté pot or rondeau, heat the extra-virgin olive oil and popcorn kernels over high heat.

Cover and let the kernels pop until the popping is very slow. Remove from the heat.

In a small sauté pan, heat the vegan butter, hot sauce, salt, red chili flakes, cayenne and lemon juice until the mixture is melted and combined.

Pour the hot sauce mixture over the popcorn and stir quickly to coat and combine.

Let cool for 5 minutes. Toss the popcorn again.

Note: 3 tablespoons (26 g) of kernels pops 7½ cups (1 kg) of popcorn. The analysis below is for 8 servings.

NUTRITION INFORMATION PER SERVING: Calories: 140, Total Fat: 10 g, Saturated Fat: 3 g, Total Carbohydrates: 11 g, Fiber: 2 g, Net Carbohydrates: 9 g, Sugar: 0 g, Protein: 2 g, Sodium: 389 mg

RAINBOW CHARD CHIPS

SERVINGS: 2

If you love the salty crunch of a potato chip, this recipe will definitely give you your fix without the guilt and spike in blood sugar. Swiss chard is high in fiber, vitamin K and alpha-linolenic acid—a type of omega-3 fatty acid that may help control blood sugar. Feel free to run with this recipe and spice these chips any way you choose. Garlic, onion and cayenne are a few good choices.

1 large bunch rainbow chard, stemmed, dried on paper towels, leaves torn into bite-size pieces (about 4 cups [1.3 kg])

Extra-virgin olive oil cooking spray

¼ tsp sea salt

Black pepper

Paprika (optional)

Preheat the oven to 250°F (121°C).

Arrange the rainbow chard in one layer on a baking sheet.

Spray the rainbow chard with 20 sprays of the extra-virgin olive oil and sprinkle with salt, black pepper and paprika, if using.

Bake for 20 minutes.

Remove from the oven. Let cool for 2 minutes.

NUTRITIONAL INFORMATION PER SERVING: Calories: 38, Total Fat: 3 g, Saturated Fat: 0 g, Total Carbohydrates: 3 g, Fiber: 1 g, Net Carbohydrates: 2 g, Sugar: 1 g, Protein: 1 g, Sodium: 450 mg

NIRVANA CHIPS

SERVINGS: 1

This healthy version of potato chips uses sweet potato, making them much more flavorful and nutritious than the original. The chips are equally as delicious on their own as when they are paired with a dip, such as the Za'atar-Flaxseed Hummus (page 131).

1 sweet potato, mandolined thinly

1 tbsp (15 ml) extra-virgin olive oil

½ tsp fresh rosemary

½ tsp salt

Preheat the oven to 350°F (177°C). Line a baking sheet with parchment paper.

Toss the sweet potatoes with the extra-virgin olive oil, rosemary and salt. Mix well to ensure that all slices are coated.

Place the sweet potatoes in one even layer on the prepared baking sheet. Bake for 10 minutes. Flip the sweet potatoes over.

Bake for another 10 to 15 minutes, or until the slices crisp up at the edges and are firm at the center.

Let cool for 5 minutes.

NUTRITIONAL INFORMATION PER SERVING: Calories: 174, Total Fat: 15.5 g, Saturated Fat: 1.9 g, Total Carbohydrates: 12 g, Fiber: 2 g, Net Carbohydrates: 10 g, Sugar: 4.2 g, Protein: 1 g, Sodium: 600 mg

GREEN VITALITY TOAST WITH CHILI-LIME SALT

SERVINGS: 1

Choosing multigrain toast in place of traditional white bread adds fiber, B vitamins and magnesium to your breakfast. Creamy avocado is the perfect spread for toast as it is full of biotin and monounsaturated fatty acids to balance out the meal's carbohydrates, for better blood sugar control.

½ avocado, cubed

2 slices multigrain bread, toasted

⅛ tsp large-flake sea salt

⅛ tsp chili powder

Zest of 1 lime, remaining lime reserved

Place the avocado in a bowl and mash with the back of a fork or a potato masher. Spread the mashed avocado over the toast.

Mix the sea salt, chili powder and lime zest in a small bowl, then sprinkle the mixture on top of the toast.

Cut the zested lime into wedges and serve with the toast.

NUTRITIONAL INFORMATION PER SERVING: Calories: 252, Total Fat: 13 g, Saturated Fat: 2 g, Total Carbohydrates: 29 g, Fiber: 9 g, Net Carbohydrates: 20 g, Sugar: 4 g, Protein: 8 g, Sodium: 511 mg

HOMEMADE STRAWBERRY ICE CREAM

SERVINGS: 2

Frozen fruits are special in that they take on a creamy consistency when blended. Strawberries and bananas work best for this, and the açai and mint paired with the strawberries in this recipe are an incredible flavor combination.

1 package frozen açai (e.g., Sambazon brand)

8 oz (227 g) frozen strawberries

4 sprigs mint, leaves only

1 cup (237 ml) unsweetened soy milk

Combine the açai, strawberries, mint and soy milk in a blender. Puree until very smooth.

Freeze immediately for at least 1 hour.

Serve frozen.

NUTRITIONAL INFORMATION PER SERVING: Calories: 213, Total Fat: 10.2 g, Saturated Fat: 1.5 g, Total Carbohydrates: 22.6 g, Fiber: 5.1 g, Net Carbohydrates: 17.5 g, Sugar: 9.8 g, Protein: 9.6 g, Sodium: 114 mg

GRANOLA CLUSTERS

SERVINGS: 4

These crunchy clusters are going to be one of your new favorite recipes. Toasted coconut flakes and bitter cacao nibs are the perfect counterpart for the naturally sweet mulberries. I love using supernutrient-dense mulberries in this recipe, as they are high in antioxidants, iron, vitamins and fiber. What does that mean for you? Better blood sugar control! These clusters are great on their own as a midday snack or dessert, or they are a fantastic addition to a bowl of yogurt and berries.

½ cup (50 g) dried mulberries

2 tbsp (9 g) coconut flakes, toasted

½ cup (40 g) rolled oats

½ cup (68 g) chopped pistachios

1 tbsp (9 g) cacao nibs

Pinch of salt

2 tsp (5 g) orange zest

1 tbsp (15 ml) extra-virgin olive oil

2 tbsp (30 ml) dark pure maple syrup or honey

Preheat the oven to 350°F (177°C).

Combine the mulberries, coconut flakes, oats, pistachios, cacao nibs, salt and orange zest in a bowl. Mix thoroughly.

Add the extra-virgin olive oil and maple syrup.

Spread the mixture in one even layer on a baking sheet and bake for 10 minutes.

Let cool for 5 minutes and break into clusters.

NUTRITIONAL INFORMATION PER SERVING: Calories: 257, Total Fat: 16 g, Saturated Fat: 5 g, Total Carbohydrates: 25 g, Fiber: 4 g, Net Carbohydrates: 21 g, Sugar: 10 g, Protein: 6 g, Sodium: 43 mg

STRAWBERRY SMOOTHIE

SERVINGS: 1

A quick and easy recipe that you can use as a breakfast or a snack, before or after the gym or to avoid that midday slump. Blend this simple smoothie and enjoy!

1 cup (151 g) strawberries

8 oz (227 g) unsweetened coconut milk yogurt

Blend the strawberries and yogurt for a delicious smoothie.

Make and chill for 1 to 2 hours before serving.

NUTRITIONAL INFORMATION PER SERVING: Calories: 235, Total Fat: 8 g, Saturated Fat: 8 g, Total Carbohydrates: 41 g, Fiber: 6 g, Net Carbohydrates: 35 g, Sugar: 33 g, Protein: 1 g, Sodium: 8 mg

PEANUT BUTTER BITES

SERVINGS: 10

When your energy starts to lag, you can count on these delicious bites to be your pick-me-up. Full of healthy fats and complex carbohydrates, these sweet and salty snacks will hit the spot and save you from your midafternoon slump. The figs and oats will give you a burst of energy, the good fats in the peanut butter, pistachios and flaxseed meal will sustain you until dinner, and the combination of sweet and savory will satisfy any craving.

½ cup (83 g) dried figs

1½ cups (121 g) rolled oats

Pinch of salt

½ cup (76 g) chopped pistachios

¼ cup (60 ml) pure maple syrup

½ cup (90 g) unsalted, creamy peanut butter

1 tbsp (10 g) flaxseed meal + 3 tbsp (45 ml) water, mixed well

Extra-virgin olive oil spray

Puree the dried figs in a food processor until they clump into a sticky ball. Place the fig puree in a bowl with the oats, salt and pistachios.

In a small saucepan, warm the maple syrup over low heat. Whisk in the peanut butter.

Add the flaxseed mixture to the fig mixture and stir in the maple syrup mixture.

Line a loaf pan with plastic wrap. Spray with extra-virgin olive oil spray.

Cover with plastic wrap (also sprayed with nonstick spray) and place in the refrigerator to chill for 30 minutes.

Remove the firmed mixture from the refrigerator and chop into bites of your desired size.

NUTRITIONAL INFORMATION PER SERVING (3 pieces): Calories: 200, Total Fat: 10 g, Saturated Fat: 1.5 g, Total Carbohydrates: 23 g, Fiber: 4 g, Net Carbohydrates: 19 g, Sugar: 7 g, Protein: 6 g, Sodium: 20 mg

ANTIOXIDANT CHOCOLATE COINS

YIELD: 24 MINI MUFFINS (COINS); SERVING SIZE: 2 COINS

Who doesn't love chocolate? Its velvety smooth texture and subtle sweetness is hard to resist, and if you have these delicious chocolate coins lying around, you don't have to! Chocolate is beaming with health benefits from heart and brain health to disease prevention; this sweet confection has even been shown to do wonders for the skin. Not only are these chocolate coins easy to make, but they taste amazing any time of the day. Enjoy two coins after dinner to satisfy your sweet tooth, or even alongside a tall glass of hemp milk for a protein-packed snack.

¼ cup (25 g) goji berries

2 tbsp (9 g) shredded coconut

2 tbsp (17 g) cacao nibs

1 cup (136 g) dark chocolate chunks

Line a 24-well mini-muffin pan with paper liners.

Sprinkle the goji berries, coconut and cacao nibs into the liners.

In a small saucepot, melt the chocolate and pour enough into each muffin well to bind the ingredients.

Let cool and harden.

NUTRITION INFORMATION PER SERVING: Calories: 136, Total Fat: 10 g, Saturated Fat: 6 g, Total Carbohydrates: 16 g, Fiber: 2 g, Net Carbohydrates: 14 g, Sugar: 10 g, Protein: 2 g, Sodium: 14 mg

APPLE CINNAMON BARS

SERVINGS: 5

When it comes to the all-American apple pie flavor, these apple cinnamon bars hit the nail on the head. Sweet cinnamon and nutmeg mixed with cloves and ginger are the perfect addition to tangy Granny Smith apples. Add some oats, almonds and flaxseeds for a dose of healthy fats and filling protein and fiber, and these bars make the perfect, nutritionally rounded meal—or on-the-go snack.

Extra-virgin olive oil spray

1 tbsp (10 g) flaxseed meal + 3 tbsp (45 ml) water, mixed well

¼ cup (25 g) almond flour

½ cup (80 g) steel-cut oats

¼ cup (43 g) finely chopped almonds

2 tbsp (43 ml) honey

¼ tsp baking powder

Pinch of salt

Pinch of ground cinnamon

Pinch of ground nutmeg

Pinch of ground cloves

Pinch of ground ginger

1 tbsp (15 ml) coconut oil

¾ cup (135 g) peeled, cored and chopped Granny Smith apple

Preheat the oven to 375°F (191°C). Lightly grease a baking sheet with the extra-virgin olive oil spray.

Combine all the remaining ingredients and mix well.

Flatten the mixture into a square on the prepared pan and bake until fully heated through, about 20 minutes.

Let cool for 5 minutes and cut into 8 equal pieces.

NUTRITIONAL INFORMATION PER SERVING: Calories: 160, Total Fat: 9 g, Saturated Fat: 3 g, Total Carbohydrates: 18 g, Fiber: 3 g, Net Carbohydrates: 15 g, Sugar: 6 g, Protein: 4 g, Sodium: 60 mg

CRUNCHY CHICKPEAS

SERVINGS: 6

There's nothing quite as satisfying as a crunchy, crispy snack when the craving hits. Luckily, these roasted chickpeas will hit the spot without all of the calories, fat and sodium of typical snack foods. They are chock-full of fiber and protein to fill you up, keep you satisfied and help stabilize your blood sugar throughout the day and are high in magnesium, which is crucial for glucose metabolism and blood sugar control.

1 (15 oz [425 g]) can garbanzo beans (chickpeas), drained, rinsed and spun dry

2 tbsp (30 ml) extra-virgin olive oil

¼ tsp salt

SPICE BLENDS

1 tbsp (6 g) Old Bay seasoning and pinch of cayenne pepper

or ½ tbsp (3 g) black pepper, ½ tablespoon (3 g) chili powder and 1 tsp (2 g) dried parsley

or 1 tsp (5 ml) pure maple syrup and 1 tbsp (6 g) pumpkin pie spice

Preheat the oven to 400°F (204°C). Line a baking sheet with parchment paper.

Lay the garbanzo beans on paper towels and pat dry again with another set of paper towels.

On the prepared baking sheet, arrange the garbanzo beans in one layer and toss with the extra-virgin olive oil and salt.

Roast for 20 minutes on the middle rack. Rotate the beans and roast for another 20 minutes, until golden brown and crunchy.

Remove from the oven and season immediately with the spice blend of your choice.

NUTRITIONAL INFORMATION PER SERVING: Calories: 160, Total Fat: 7 g, Saturated Fat: 1 g, Total Carbohydrates: 19 g, Fiber: 5 g, Net Carbohydrates: 14 g, Sugar: 0 g, Protein: 6 g, Sodium: 100 mg

NOTE: Old Bay and cayenne adds 0 mg Sodium; pepper, chili powder and parsley adds 2 g Carbohydrates, 2 g Fiber, 10 mg Sodium; maple syrup and pumpkin pie spice adds 10 Calories, 1 g Fiber, 1 g Sugar, 5 mg Sodium.

CHAPTER 11

VEGGIES

Often, vegetables get a bad rap. But, really, is there anything better than vegetables? They are nature's perfect food and my favorite food. They are low in calories, high in fiber, nutrients and antioxidants, colorful and, when prepared in the right way, taste amazing. Plus, they are really easy and quick to make!

Whether I am cooking favorites, such as my Spicy Ginger Baby Bok Choy (page 155), Rosemary Roasted Root Vegetables (page 156) or the ever-favorite Creamy Cauliflower Mashed Potatoes (page 158)—all the flavor, half the fat—or introducing something new, such as Sautéed Tuscan Kale (page 152), I know my clients will love every last bite. In fact, when I recommend these recipes to my die-hard omnivore clients, they can't believe how good they taste.

If you're new to vegetables, don't be afraid to experiment—you can almost never go wrong. My Italian side says just add garlic and olive oil and a few seasonings, such as oregano or parsley, and everything tastes great! Feel free to increase or decrease the ingredients in these recipes to suit your family's preferences, as they can be made many different ways. Vegetables are so versatile and easy to prepare, you can feel confident making them in a variety of ways.

GLOWING GREEN SEAWEED SALAD

SERVINGS: 2

A seaweed salad offers variety from your more traditional salads while providing a host of nutritional benefits. Seaweed is high in protein and minerals especially iodine, calcium, iron and magnesium. It also is high in vitamin C and contains many anti-inflammatory properties. Eat up!

1 oz (28 g) dried seaweed (any kind)

Water

1 tbsp (15 ml) rice vinegar

1 tbsp (15 ml) sesame oil

1 tbsp (15 ml) soy sauce, tamari or liquid aminos

2 tsp (10 ml) agave nectar

½ tsp salt

¼ tsp ginger, grated

1 tsp (3 g) white sesame seeds, toasted

1 scallion, minced

Place the seaweed in water. Soak for 10 minutes to rehydrate.

Combine all the other ingredients, except the sesame seeds and scallion, and whisk together.

Drain the seaweed and squeeze out any excess water, using a towel. Cut into thin strips.

Toss the seaweed with the dressing. Sprinkle with the sesame seeds and scallion.

NUTRITIONAL INFORMATION PER SERVING: Calories: 141, Total Fat: 7.6 g, Saturated Fat: 1.1 g, Total Carbohydrates: 14.7 g, Fiber: 5.9 g, Net Carbohydrates: 8.8 g, Sugar: 7.9 g, Protein: 2.2 g, Sodium: 608 mg

COOLING CUCUMBER SALAD

SERVINGS: 2

Cucumber salad is the perfect side to any meal. This light recipe is both hydrating and nourishing. Choosing sesame oil instead of traditional canola oil adds a toasty flavor along with heart-healthy unsaturated fats and omega-3 fatty acids.

2 Japanese or Persian cucumbers, sliced thinly on a bias

Salt

½ tsp sesame oil

1 tsp (5 ml) soy sauce

½ tsp mirin

1 tsp (1 g) very thinly sliced scallion

Toss the cucumbers thoroughly with salt and place in a colander in the sink.

Let them sit for 10 minutes.

Rinse the cucumbers with water and spin dry. Toss the cucumbers with the remaining ingredients.

NUTRITIONAL INFORMATION PER SERVING: Calories: 62, Total Fat: 1 g, Saturated Fat: 0 g, Total Carbohydrates: 12 g, Fiber: 2 g, Net Carbohydrates: 10 g, Sugar: 6 g, Protein: 2 g, Sodium: 521 mg

LEMONY BRUSSELS SPROUTS

SERVINGS: 1

Lemon is a lovely way to cut the sharp flavor normally associated with Brussels sprouts, and cooking them in boiling water first instead of entirely in the pan gets them finished much more quickly.

Water

Salt

6 oz (170 g) Brussels sprouts, washed

1 tbsp (15 ml) extra-virgin olive oil

1 oz (20 g) yellow onion, minced

1 clove garlic, minced

1 Meyer lemon, quartered

Black pepper (optional)

Red pepper flakes (optional)

Bring a medium stockpot of lightly salted water to a rolling boil.

Add the Brussels sprouts and blanch for 1 to 2 minutes. Test one for tenderness; it should be al dente.

Shock immediately in ice water for 2 to 3 minutes. Strain the Brussels sprouts and spin dry.

In a medium sauté pan, heat the extra-virgin olive oil over medium heat. Add the onion, garlic and a pinch of salt. Sauté for 1 minute.

Increase the heat to high. Add the Brussels sprouts and a pinch of salt. Sauté for 4 to 5 minutes. Remove from the heat.

Squeeze 2 wedges of Meyer lemon, through a small strainer, over the Brussels sprouts and stir to combine.

Season with black pepper and red pepper flakes, if desired.

Add additional squeezes of Meyer lemon, if desired.

NUTRITIONAL INFORMATION PER SERVING: Calories: 230, Total Fat: 15.5 g, Saturated Fat: 1.1 g, Total Carbohydrates: 22.2 g, Fiber: 9.6 g, Net Carbohydrates: 12.6 g, Sugar: 6.7 g, Protein: 7.9 g, Sodium: 45.5 mg

SAUTÉED TUSCAN KALE

SERVINGS: 2

Kale is an extremely nutrient-rich green vegetable, and it is great to collect as many ways to cook it as possible. As is the case with this recipe, sometimes the simplest preparations are the most delicious!

2 tsp (10 ml) walnut oil

1 oz (28 g) yellow onion, sliced

½ tsp balsamic vinegar

4 oz (113 g) Tuscan kale, ribs removed, chopped

Salt

Black pepper

In a medium sauté pan, heat the walnut oil over medium heat until slick and shiny.

Lower the heat to low. Add the onion and balsamic vinegar and sauté for 15 minutes, until lightly caramelized.

Increase the heat to medium.

Add the kale and sauté for another 4 to 5 minutes, until the kale is dark green and begins to wilt slightly.

Season with salt and black pepper to taste.

NUTRITIONAL INFORMATION PER SERVING: Calories: 75, Total Fat: 5.1 g, Saturated Fat: 0.6 g, Total Carbohydrates: 6.8 g, Fiber: 1.6 g, Net Carbohydrates: 5.2 g, Sugar: 1.2 g, Protein: 2.4 g, Sodium: 24.9 mg

ISRAELI SALAD

SERVINGS: 4

This salad is a fantastically fresh start to any meal. The bright colors of the veggies are as beautiful as the tangy lemon dressing is simple. All you have to do here is toss everything together and you have a dish to impress! You can have it as an entrée if you add baked falafel, as a side dish or as a starter.

6 oz (170 g) Japanese or Persian cucumber, diced

4 oz (113 g) Roma tomato, seeded and diced

2 oz (57 g) red bell pepper, diced

2 tbsp (5 g) fresh parsley, chopped

1 scallion, minced

Juice of ½ lemon

Pinch of dried oregano

Salt and black pepper

Combine the cucumber, tomato, bell pepper, parsley, scallion and lemon juice.

Season with the oregano and salt and black pepper to taste.

NUTRITIONAL INFORMATION PER SERVING: Calories: 23, Total Fat: 0.1 g, Saturated Fat: 0 g, Total Carbohydrates: 4.8 g, Fiber: 1.6 g, Net Carbohydrates: 3.2 g, Sugar: 1.6 g, Protein: 0.6 g, Sodium: 0 mg

WILTED SPINACH
WITH ROASTED PEARS AND WALNUTS

SERVINGS: 2

The pear in this recipe provides the perfect counterpoint of sweetness to an otherwise savory dish. Prepare to amaze your guests by serving this as a starter at your next dinner!

1 pear, peeled, cored and diced

2 tsp (10 ml) extra-virgin olive oil

1 scallion, sliced thinly

¼ cup (85 g) fennel, mandolined

4 cups (1.3 kg) fresh spinach

Juice of ¼ lemon

½ tsp whole-grain mustard

⅛ tsp salt

Black pepper

¼ cup (30 g) walnuts, chopped and toasted

Preheat the oven to 400°F (204°C). Line a baking sheet with parchment paper.

Place the pear slices on the prepared baking sheet. Roast for about 20 minutes, flipping once, until all sides are lightly browned. Set aside to cool.

Meanwhile, heat 1 teaspoon (5 ml) of the extra-virgin olive oil in a small pan over medium heat.

Add the scallion, fennel and spinach and cook for 2 to 3 minutes, until the spinach is wilted.

In a small bowl, whisk together the lemon juice, mustard, remaining 1 teaspoon (5 ml) of extra-virgin olive oil, salt and black pepper to taste.

Top the spinach mixture with the pears, walnuts and dressing.

NUTRITIONAL INFORMATION PER SERVING: Calories: 194, Total Fat: 14.9 g, Saturated Fat: 1.7 g, Total Carbohydrates: 13.2 g, Fiber: 4 g, Net Carbohydrates: 9.2 g, Sugar: 7.2 g, Protein: 4.6 g, Sodium: 64.7 mg

SPICY GINGER BABY BOK CHOY

SERVINGS: 2

Baby bok choy is actually a member of the cabbage family that has been cultivated by the Chinese for over 5,000 years! This crisp veggie boasts a full day's worth of vitamin A and nearly a day's worth of vitamin C. Enjoy this as a satisfying side dish, or add tofu, bell pepper, scallions and broccoli for a satisfying stir-fry.

1 tsp (5 ml) extra-virgin olive oil

1 tsp (5 ml) sesame oil

10 oz (284 g) baby bok choy, washed and spun dry

2 tsp (10 g) minced fresh ginger

1 clove garlic, minced

2 tsp (10 ml) soy sauce

Pinch of wasabi powder (optional)

Heat the extra-virgin olive oil and sesame oil in large sauté pan until slick and shiny.

Add the bok choy, ginger, garlic, soy sauce and wasabi powder, if using.

Sauté for 3 to 4 minutes, until the bok choy leaves are bright green and the stems are soft.

NUTRITIONAL INFORMATION PER SERVING: Calories: 67, Total Fat: 5 g, Saturated Fat: 1 g, Total Carbohydrates: 5 g, Fiber: 2 g, Net Carbohydrates: 3 g, Sugar: 2 g, Protein: 3 g, Sodium: 237 mg

ROSEMARY ROASTED ROOT VEGETABLES

SERVINGS: 2

There is something about the bright orange color and fragrant rosemary in this dish that take me back to a holiday table—so comforting. Sweet potatoes are the perfect alternative to white potatoes as they are full of vitamins, minerals and fiber, which delays the release of sugar into the blood. This hearty mixture goes perfectly alongside a peppery arugula and white bean salad dressed simply with lemon juice and extra-virgin olive oil.

1 sweet potato, peeled and diced

2 parsnips, peeled and diced

1 acorn squash, seeded, then cut into half-moons

1 tbsp (15 ml) extra-virgin olive oil

½ tsp salt

¼ tsp black pepper

1 tsp (1 g) fresh rosemary, minced

Preheat the oven to 375°F (191°C).

Toss all the ingredients together in a large bowl.

Arrange the mixture in a single layer on a sheet pan.

Bake for 30 to 40 minutes, until the sweet potato can be pierced easily by a fork.

Let cool for 5 minutes.

NUTRITIONAL INFORMATION PER SERVING: Calories: 316, Total Fat: 8 g, Saturated Fat: 1 g, Total Carbohydrates: 63 g, Fiber: 11 g, Net Carbohydrates: 52 g, Sugar: 10 g, Protein: 5 g, Sodium: 604 mg

SESAME TAMARI EDAMAME AND SHIITAKE MUSHROOMS

SERVINGS: 2

This flavorful side dish is the perfect accompaniment to grilled tofu or noodle salad. Edamame beans are great served alongside almost any meal, and they are easily purchased already shelled and frozen, requiring only a few minutes to prepare.

1 (8 oz [227 g]) package frozen edamame

1 tsp (5 g) sesame oil

8 oz (227 g) shiitake mushrooms, stemmed and sliced

¼ tsp fresh ginger, grated

2 tsp (10 ml) low-sodium tamari or liquid aminos

2 scallions, sliced thinly

1 tsp (3 g) black sesame seeds

Bring a large pot of water to a rolling boil.

Add the frozen edamame and cook for 2 to 3 minutes.

Strain and rinse the edamame in cold water for 30 seconds. Set aside.

In a large sauté pan, heat the sesame oil until slick and shiny.

Add the shiitake mushrooms, ginger and tamari. Sauté for 3 to 4 minutes, until the shiitakes reduce in size by about half.

Add the edamame and sauté for another minute.

Remove from the heat and sprinkle with the scallions and sesame seeds.

NUTRITIONAL INFORMATION PER SERVING: Calories: 380, Total Fat: 17.2 g, Saturated Fat: 3 g, Total Carbohydrates: 39.3 g, Fiber: 22.1 g, Net Carbohydrates: 17.1 g, Sugar: 9.6 g, Protein: 24.3 g, Sodium: 603 mg

CREAMY CAULIFLOWER MASHED POTATOES

SERVINGS: 2

Mashed potatoes are a traditional side dish often thought of as a no-no because they are high in fat, carbs and calories. Swap out the traditional white potatoes for nutrient-dense cauliflower, and this becomes a YES! Adding roasted garlic and chives makes this mash taste divine, while nutritional yeast adds loads of B vitamins and a cheesy flavor. Use this mash in place of mashed potatoes in any meal, or try using it as a bed for your favorite vegetable chili or stewed tomatoes and chickpeas for a hearty meal that won't disappoint.

1 tsp (5 ml) extra-virgin olive oil, plus more to coat the garlic

1 head garlic, skin on

1 small head cauliflower, cored and chopped roughly

1 tbsp (15 g) vegan butter, at room temperature

2 cloves garlic, roasted

1 tsp (3 g) nutritional yeast

1 tsp (1 g) minced fresh chives

2 tbsp (30 ml) unsweetened soy creamer

Salt and black pepper

Preheat the oven to 400°F (204°C).

Coat the garlic head with extra-virgin olive oil and roast for 10 minutes. The garlic should easily slide out of the skin when done.

Boil or steam the cauliflower until very tender. Puree the cauliflower in a food processor.

Add all the other ingredients, including the remaining 1 teaspoon (5 ml) of extra-virgin olive oil, except the creamer, salt and pepper, to the processor and puree again. Add the creamer to the processor while it is still running.

Season with salt and black pepper to taste.

NUTRITION INFORMATION PER SERVING: Calories: 134, Total Fat: 10 g, Saturated Fat: 4 g, Total Carbohydrates: 8 g, Fiber: 3 g, Net Carbohydrates: 5 g, Sugar: 3 g, Protein: 5 g, Sodium: 241 mg

CHAPTER 12

STAPLES

The recipes in this chapter are an essential part of the BSM plan. When made ahead of time, they will save you a lot of time. Many of them can be prepared and either stored in the fridge for up to a week or frozen for a longer period.

Making these staples is essential because many of the products on the market are laden with sugar, salt, fat and calories. There have been so many times that I have been in the supermarket looking for a quick and easy marinara sauce to use for a last-minute dinner with friends and it has taken me an hour to find a product that didn't contain too much sugar or salt. My Vegetable Marinara Sauce (page 117) is a perfect solution for that. I include some products (pages 174–178) already vetted by me that you can keep in your pantry to help you out in a pinch.

Many of the staple recipes can be used interchangeably or, once prepared, can last for several days. For instance, once you make a batch of Lovely Lentils (page 168) you can have them as a side dish at dinner, as a soup the next day at lunch—just add some Nourishing Vegetable Broth (page 161)—or incorporate them into a salad for dinner the next night. Feel free to make a batch of Overnight Oats (page 169) to save you time in the morning. And the Daily Detox Elixir (page 160) should be consumed at the start of each day.

DAILY DETOX ELIXIR

SERVINGS: 2

Turmeric is mostly seen in its powdered form on grocery store shelves, but the fresh root version is not difficult to come across in health food stores. Combined with the ginger, the turmeric has a warming effect on the body and also helps increase your system's ability to eliminate toxins.

5 oz (142 g) fresh ginger, unpeeled, washed

5 oz (142 g) fresh turmeric, unpeeled, washed

½ fresh lemon, squeezed

8 oz (227 ml) water

6 ice cubes

Juice the ginger and turmeric. You should have about 5 ounces (140 ml) of juice.

Add the lemon to the mixture and whisk thoroughly to combine.

Mix with the water and divide between 2 glasses. Add the ice.

NUTRITIONAL INFORMATION PER SERVING: Calories: 0, Total Fat: 0 g, Saturated Fat: 0 g, Total Carbohydrates: 0 g, Fiber: 0 g, Net Carbohydrates: 0 g, Sugar: 0 g, Protein: 0 g, Sodium: 0 mg

NOURISHING VEGETABLE BROTH

YIELD: 1 QUART (1 L); SERVINGS: SERVING SIZE: 1 CUP (237 ML)

This warming broth is the perfect way to add vitamins and minerals into your day. Mushrooms provide a deep, hearty aroma along with a daily dose of biotin and B vitamins, which give the body energy as they assist in the breakdown of protein, fat and carbohydrates. Use this broth as a base for many soups and side dishes. I use this vegetable broth when sautéing vegetables because it provides flavor and liquid without all of the added calories from the oil that is traditionally used in sautéing.

1 tsp (5 ml) extra-virgin olive oil

2 cloves garlic, sliced

8 oz (227 g) yellow onion, diced

4 oz (113 g) chopped celery

4 oz (113 g) chopped carrot

Pinch of salt

1 tbsp (15 ml) white wine

4 oz (113 g) cremini mushrooms, sliced

1 sprig rosemary

1 sprig thyme

2 quarts (1.8 L) cold water

Black pepper

In a medium stockpot, heat the extra-virgin olive oil over medium heat.

Add the garlic, onion, celery, carrot and salt and sauté for 4 to 5 minutes. Add the wine and sauté for 1 minute, until the wine has been absorbed. Add the mushrooms, rosemary and thyme and sauté for 2 minutes.

Add the cold water and bring to a very light simmer.

Let simmer for 4 to 6 hours, skimming the top of any scum that forms.

Strain. Add black pepper to taste.

NUTRITIONAL INFORMATION PER SERVING: Calories: 60.8, Total Fat: 1.5 g, Saturated Fat: 0.3 g, Total Carbohydrates: 10.5 g, Fiber: 2.8 g, Net Carbohydrates: 7.8 g, Sugar: 5 g, Protein: 1.8 g, Sodium: 47.5 mg

DRESSINGS

Commercially prepared salad dressings are one of the most deceitful products on the market, as they are generally laden with sugar, fat, sodium and preservatives. The salad dressings here are so easy to make they will leave you wondering why you ever bought store-bought dressings in the first place. They taste delicious, are nutritious and complement any salad they are topping—depending on your mood. If you feel like having some spice that day, try the Jalapeño Lime Vinaigrette. Feeling like taking a trip to the Middle East? Go for the Light Tahini Dressing—not just for salads—also a great marinade. The Dijon Vinaigrette goes with just about anything! The Pomegranate Vinaigrette tastes especially great on a warm summer day, while I like to have the Sesame Ginger Dressing when I am in the mood for an Asian flair. Make a batch of your favorite and have it on hand for the week.

JALAPEÑO LIME VINAIGRETTE

SERVINGS: 2

1 tbsp (15 ml) extra-virgin olive oil

Juice of 1 lime

2 tsp (10 ml) whole-grain mustard

1 small jalapeño chile, seeded, deveined and minced

1 tbsp (3 g) chopped fresh cilantro

Pinch of salt

1 tbsp (21 ml) honey

Whisk together the extra-virgin olive oil, lime juice, mustard, jalapeño, cilantro, salt and honey in a bowl.

NUTRITIONAL INFORMATION PER SERVING: Calories: 101, Total Fat: 7 g, Saturated Fat: 1 g, Total Carbohydrates: 11 g, Fiber: 0 g, Net Carbohydrates: 11 g, Sugar: 9 g, Protein: 0 g, Sodium: 60 mg

POMEGRANATE VINAIGRETTE

SERVINGS: 4

¼ cup (50 g) pomegranate arils

2 tbsp (30 ml) balsamic vinegar

1 tbsp (15 ml) extra-virgin olive oil

2 tsp (11 ml) Dijon mustard

Salt and black pepper

In a small bowl, mash the pomegranate arils to make pomegranate juice. They should yield about 3 tablespoons (45 ml) of juice. Discard the pomegranate pulp.

Whisk together the rest of the ingredients with the pomegranate juice, adding salt and black pepper to taste. Alternatively, put all the ingredients in a small jar with a tight-fitting lid and shake well.

NUTRITIONAL INFORMATION PER SERVING: Calories: 151, Total Fat: 14 g, Saturated Fat: 2 g, Total Carbohydrates: 6 g, Fiber: 0 g, Net Carbohydrates: 6 g, Sugar: 5 g, Protein: 0 g, Sodium: 126 mg

DIJON VINAIGRETTE

SERVINGS: 2

2 cloves garlic, minced

1½ tsp (8 ml) Dijon mustard

1 tbsp (15 ml) lemon juice, or to taste

3 tbsp (45 ml) extra-virgin olive oil

Salt and black pepper

Place the garlic, mustard, lemon juice and extra-virgin olive oil in a small jar.

Season with salt and black pepper to taste.

Shake the jar to combine. Serve.

NUTRITIONAL INFORMATION PER SERVING: Calories: 189, Total Fat: 20 g, Saturated Fat: 3 g, Total Carbohydrates: 2 g, Fiber: 0 g, Net Carbohydrates: 2 g, Sugar: 0 g, Protein: 0 g, Sodium: 91 mg

LIGHT TAHINI DRESSING

SERVINGS: 8

½ cup (115 g) tahini

½ cup (118 ml) water

1 oz (28 g) cucumber, peeled, cored and chopped

Juice of 1 lemon

1 clove garlic, minced

1 tbsp (15 ml) extra-virgin olive oil

1 tsp (5 g) salt

Pinch of black pepper

Pinch of red pepper flakes

In a medium bowl, whisk together all the ingredients.

NUTRITIONAL INFORMATION PER SERVING: Calories: 106, Total Fat: 10 g, Saturated Fat: 1 g, Total Carbohydrates: 4 g, Fiber: 1 g, Net Carbohydrates: 3 g, Sugar: 2 g, Protein: 3 g, Sodium: 300 mg

CITRUS-WALNUT DRESSING

SERVINGS: 1

Juice of 1 small lemon

¼ cup (60 ml) walnut oil

½ tsp (3 ml) Dijon mustard

½ tsp (3 g) salt

Pinch of black pepper

In a small bowl, whisk together all the ingredients.

NUTRITION INFORMATION PER SERVING: Calories: 124, Total Fat: 14 g, Saturated Fat: 1 g, Total Carbohydrates: 1 g, Fiber: 0 g, Net Carbohydrates: 1 g, Sugar: 0 g, Protein: 0 g, Sodium: 310 mg

SESAME GINGER DRESSING

SERVINGS: 4

1 tsp (5 g) fresh ginger, grated

1 clove garlic, minced

1 tsp (5 ml) sesame oil

¼ cup (60 ml) peanut oil

Juice of 1 lime

½ tsp black or white sesame seeds

In a small bowl, whisk together all the ingredients until well emulsified, or place in small mason jar and shake vigorously.

NUTRITIONAL INFORMATION PER SERVING: Calories: 135, Total Fat: 15 g, Saturated Fat: 2 g, Total Carbohydrates: 1 g, Fiber: 0 g, Net Carbohydrates: 1 g, Sugar: 0 g, Protein: 0 g, Sodium: 1 mg

DAILY FOUNDATIONAL VEGETABLES

SERVINGS: 2

Coconut oil is a great go-to for frying veggies because it can withstand a higher temperature than other fats can, such as extra-virgin olive oil. The vegetables suggested in this recipe pair together deliciously, but feel free to substitute your favorites as well. These vegetables are great served over brown rice or lentils.

1 tbsp (15 ml) coconut oil

½ yellow onion, sliced

½ cup (76 g) cremini mushrooms, sliced

1 large red bell pepper, julienned

1 cup (151 g) baby zucchini, sliced lengthwise

2 cups (681 g) fresh spinach

Salt and black pepper

Heat the coconut oil in a medium skillet over medium-high heat.

Sauté the onion and mushrooms for 2 to 3 minutes. Add the bell pepper and zucchini and cook for 4 to 5 minutes. Add the spinach and cook for 1 to 2 minutes, until the spinach wilts.

Season with salt and black pepper to taste.

Serve immediately.

NUTRITIONAL INFORMATION PER SERVING: Calories: 124, Total Fat: 7.3 g, Saturated Fat: 6.1 g, Total Carbohydrates: 12.6 g, Fiber: 4 g, Net Carbohydrates: 8.6 g, Sugar: 6.2 g, Protein: 4 g, Sodium: 100 mg

LOVELY LENTILS

SERVINGS: 4

This recipe is a great staple to have in your arsenal—all of the ingredients are easily on hand in your kitchen, and the end result is so versatile that it can be enjoyed on its own, or you can get creative and add your favorite seasonings, such as cumin or fresh cilantro.

1 cup (201 g) dried green lentils

2 cups (473 ml) water, plus more if needed

1 tsp (5 g) salt

1 clove garlic, crushed

2 oz (57 g) onion, roughly chopped

Bring the lentils, water, salt, garlic and onion to a boil.

Lower the heat to a light simmer and cook, uncovered, for about 20 minutes, until the lentils are tender to the bite. Add more water if needed.

Strain. Pick out the garlic and onion.

NUTRITIONAL INFORMATION PER SERVING: Calories: 77, Total Fat: 0 g, Saturated Fat: 0 g, Total Carbohydrates: 20.4 g, Fiber: 9.2 g, Net Carbohydrates: 11.2 g, Sugar: 0.6 g, Protein: 8.2 g, Sodium: 6 mg

OVERNIGHT OATS

SERVINGS: 4

Steel-cut oats are more nutritious than quick-cooking oats due to their higher fiber content. This means their sugars are absorbed more slowly into the bloodstream. In addition, they are less processed than rolled oats, which have been steamed and roasted prior to making their way to the supermarket shelves. Cooking this whole grain overnight means you can have a hearty, healthy breakfast in no time. Try topping with blueberries, cinnamon and slivered almonds for a delicious treat.

4 cups (946 ml) filtered water

1 cup (161 g) steel-cut oats

¼ tsp salt

Your choice of toppings: blueberries, apples, raspberries, banana, peanut butter, walnuts, pistachios and/or cinnamon

Pour the water into a Dutch oven or large saucepan and bring to a rapid boil over high heat.

Pour the oats and salt into the water and stir for 1 minute.

Turn off the heat and cover. Let sit overnight.

The next day, uncover and heat the oats over medium heat, stirring, until heated through.

Serve with your favorite toppings.

NUTRITIONAL INFORMATION PER SERVING: Calories: 170, Total Fat: 3 g, Saturated Fat: 1 g, Total Carbohydrates: 29 g, Fiber: 5 g, Net Carbohydrates: 25 g, Sugar: 0 g, Protein: 7 g, Sodium: 147 mg

KITCHEN SINK FRUIT COMPOTE

SERVINGS: 2

Canned pie fillings and fruit compotes are full of sugar, preservatives and artificial coloring. This fresh alternative not only counts as a serving of fruit, but can be enjoyed any time of the day. Chia seeds act as a natural thickening agent, as they form a gelatinous consistency when placed in liquid. Try substituting chia seeds for cornstarch in any recipe for added nutrition. These seeds are a true powerhouse and are considered one of the highest plant-based sources of fiber, protein and omega-3 fatty acids.

½ cup (118 ml) water

¼ cup (60 ml) organic orange juice

¼ cup (40 g) chia seeds

½ tsp lemon zest

½ cup (76 g) strawberries

½ cup (68 g) raspberries

In a small pot over low heat, combine the water, orange juice and chia seeds. Heat, stirring well, for 2 to 3 minutes.

Add the lemon zest, strawberries and raspberries and cook for 5 minutes.

Remove from the heat and let cool.

Serve with your favorite breakfast cereal or dessert.

NUTRITIONAL INFORMATION PER SERVING: Calories: 111.5, Total Fat: 4.5 g, Saturated Fat: 0.5 g, Total Carbohydrates: 16 g, Fiber: 7.5 g, Net Carbohydrates: 8.5 g, Sugar: 6 g, Protein: 3 g, Sodium: 3.5 mg

CASHEW DREAM CHEESE

SERVINGS: 16

Soaked nuts create a very creamy spread when blended, and this recipe mimics traditional cream cheese incredibly well with the rich flavor of the tahini and the sour lemon juice. This spread is a great addition to breakfast, lunch or a snack in between!

1 cup (111 g) cashews, soaked overnight, drained and rinsed

1 tbsp (9 g) nutritional yeast

1 tsp (5 g) salt

Juice of 1 lemon

½ tsp tahini

2 tbsp (30 ml) cold water

Combine all the ingredients in a blender and puree until very, very fine.

NUTRITIONAL INFORMATION PER SERVING: Calories: 42, Total Fat: 3 g, Saturated Fat: 0.5 g, Total Carbohydrates: 2.6 g, Fiber: 0.3 g, Net Carbohydrates: 2.3 g, Sugar: 0.5 g, Protein: 1.5 g, Sodium: 0 mg

VEGETABLE MARINARA SAUCE

SERVINGS: 15

Marinara sauce is a great low-calorie and low-carbohydrate way to sneak in more veggies; ½ cup (120 ml) of marinara sauce counts as one serving of veggies! However, most store-bought brands contain added sugar and are high in sodium. Use this tasty homemade marinara sauce to spice up your favorite foods—pour it over steamed broccoli, mix it in with sautéed mushrooms or even use it as a base for a homemade soup!

2 tbsp (30 ml) extra-virgin olive oil

2 or 3 cloves garlic, minced

1 (28 oz [794 g]) can whole San Marzano tomatoes

⅓ cup (12 g) chopped fresh parsley, or ¼ cup (7 g) dried

1 bay leaf

Salt

Red pepper flakes (optional)

Coat a saucepan with extra-virgin olive oil.

Add the garlic to the pan and sauté over medium-low heat until golden brown, about 1 minute (don't allow to burn).

Add the tomatoes, parsley, bay leaf and a pinch of salt.

Bring up to gentle boil, then with a potato masher, mash the tomatoes until you can't see any big chunks.

Lower the heat to medium and simmer for 20 to 30 minutes.

Add red pepper flakes, if desired. Remove and discard the bay leaf.

NUTRITIONAL INFORMATION PER SERVING: Calories: 30, Total Fat: 2 g, Saturated Fat: 0 g, Total Carbohydrates: 2 g, Fiber: 1 g, Net Carbohydrates: 1 g, Sugar: 1 g, Protein: 0 g, Sodium: 95 mg

RESOURCES

Definitions

A1c: A blood test (also known as glycated hemoglobin, glycosylated hemoglobin, hemoglobin A1c and HbA1c) used to diagnose type 1 and type 2 diabetes. The A1c test reflects your average blood sugar level for the past two to three months. The higher the A1c level, the poorer your blood sugar control and the higher your risk of diabetes complications.

Blood sugar: The amount of sugar present in the blood. A normal level is less than 100 mg/dl in a fasting state (eight hours without eating) and less than 140 mg/dl two hours after eating.

Carbohydrate counting: Carbohydrate counting is a meal planning tool for use in managing blood sugar levels. It can be used in many situations: prediabetes, gestational diabetes, type 1 and type 2 diabetes and even for weight loss. A specific amount of carb is set per meal; when you count the grams of carbs, it helps you keep track of the amount of carbohydrate you are eating in that meal or snack.

Dietary fiber: Dietary fiber includes all parts of plant foods that our bodies cannot digest or absorb. Although we cannot digest dietary fiber, it provides a number of health benefits. Fiber is classified as soluble or insoluble. Insoluble fiber adds bulk to stools and promotes regular bowel movements. Soluble fiber dissolves in water and can help to lower cholesterol and blood sugar levels.

Glycemic index: A measure of how a carbohydrate containing food raises blood sugar. Foods are ranked compared to a reference food—either glucose or white bread.

Glycemic Load: A part of the glycemic index system, glycemic load is a number that estimates how much the food will raise a person's blood sugar after eating it. It is defined as the available grams of carbohydrate times the glycemic index.

Net carbohydrate: The carbohydrate that remains after the fiber is subtracted from the total grams of carbohydrate.

Sugar alcohols: Sugar alcohols are used by the food industry to add sweetness to foods without adding calories. It is unclear the extent to which they affect blood sugar.

Total grams of carbohydrate: When looking at a food label, you must look at the serving size and the total grams of carbohydrate. The total grams listed is what is contained in that serving size. It includes sugar, starch and fiber.

Guide to Approved List of BSM Foods

Make your own meals using this simple guide!

CATEGORY	FOOD ITEM	SERVING SIZE	FAT (G)	PROTEIN (G)	CARBS (G)	FIBER (G)	SODIUM (MG)	CHOLESTEROL (MG)
Beans (canned)	Eden Organic Black Beans	¼ cup (50 g)	0.5	11	29	16	10	0
	Eden Organic Garbanzo Beans	¼ cup (50 g)	2	9	28	12	10	0
	Eden Organic Green Lentils	¼ cup (50 g)	1	11	30	12	10	0
	Eden Organic Kidney Beans	¼ cup (50 g)	1	10	26	13	10	0
	Eden Organic Navy Beans	¼ cup (50 g)	0.5	9	28	12	10	0
	Eden Organic Pinto Beans	¼ cup (50 g)	0.5	8	26	11	5	0
Beans (dried)	Bob's Red Mill Lentils	¼ cup (50 g)	0.5	11	32	19	0	0
	Whole Foods bulk yellow soybeans	¼ cup (50 g)	9	17	14	8	0	0
Beverages	Almond Breeze Unsweetened Almond Milk	1 cup (237 ml)	2.5	1	2	1	180	0
	Ito En Tea's Tea Jasmine Flavor	1 cup (237 ml)	0	0	0	0	30 mg	0
	Ito En Tea's Tea Original Green Tea	1 cup (237 ml)	0	0	0	0	30 mg	0
	Numi Tea's Organic Fair Trade Breakfast Blend Tea	1 cup (237 ml)	0	0	0	0	0	0
	Numi Tea's Organic Jasmine Green Tea	1 cup (237 ml)	0	0	0	0	0	0
	San Pellegrino water	1 cup (237 ml)	0	0	0	0	10 mg	0

CATEGORY	FOOD ITEM	SERVING SIZE	FAT (G)	PROTEIN (G)	CARBS (G)	FIBER (G)	SODIUM (MG)	CHOLESTEROL (MG)
Breads and cereals	Bob's Red Mill buckwheat groats	¼ cup (40 g) dry	1	6	32	1	0	0
	Bob's Red Mill Corn Grits/ Polenta	¼ cup (40 g) dry	0.5	3	27	2	0	0
	Bob's Red Mill Hulled Millet	¼ (40 g) cup	2	7	40	4	0	0
	Bob's Red Mill Steel Cut Oats	¼ cup (40 g) dry	3	7	29	5	0	0
	Engine 2 Original Crispbread	1 piece	2.5	3	13	3	110	0
	Engine 2 Seeds and Spice Crispbread	1 piece	3	3	12	3	105	0
	Engine 2 Triple Seed Crispbread	1 piece	3.5	3	11	4	100	0
	Ezekiel 4:9 Almond Sprouted Whole Grain Cereal	½ cup (80 g)	3	8	38	6	190	0
	Ezekiel 4:9 Flax Sprouted Grain Bread	1 slice	1	5	14	4	70	0
	Ezekiel 4:9 Taco Size Whole Grain Tortilla	1 tortilla	1	3	14	2	80	0
	FiberRich+ Bran Crispbread	2 pieces	2	3	12	7	0	0
	Finn Crisp Thin Rye Crispbread	2 pieces	0	1	10	2	85	0
	GG Scandinavian Bran Crispbread	2 pieces	1	3	15	8	80	0
	GG Scandinavian Fiber Sprinkles	3 tbsp (30 g)	0	1	7	5	30	0
	Healthy Joy Bakes Omega Power Bread	1 slice	2.5	9	5	4	20	0
	John Mccann's Irish Oatmeal	¼ cup (40 g)	2.5	4	27	3	0	0
	Linwoods Ground Flax, Sesame, Pumpkin & Sesame Seeds & Goji Berries	4 tbsp (25 g)	12	6	10	8	10	0
	Wasa Fiber Crispbread	2 slices	1.5	3	14	5	100	0
Condiments and dressings	Bragg Liquid Aminos	½ tsp	0	310 mg	100 mg	0	160	0
	Bragg Apple Cider Vinegar	1 tbsp (15 ml)	0	0	0	0	0	0
	Mina Harissa Spicy Red Pepper Sauce	2 tbsp (30 ml)	1	0	2	1	1	0
	Tessemae's Balsamic Dressing	1 tbsp (15 ml)	11	0	0	0	60	0
	Tessemae's Hot Sauce	1 tbsp (15 ml)	6	0	<1	0	200	0
	Tessemae's Italian Dressing	1 tbsp (15 ml)	9	0	0	0	70	0
	Tessemae's Lemon Garlic Dressing	1 tbsp (15 ml)	12	0	0.5	0	65	0
	Tessemae's Soy Ginger Dressing	1 tbsp (15 ml)	10	0	0	0	125	0
	Tostitos Chunky Salsa, mild, medium, hot	2 tbsp (20 g)	0	0	2	0	250	0

(continued)

CATEGORY	FOOD ITEM	SERVING SIZE	FAT (G)	PROTEIN (G)	CARBS (G)	FIBER (G)	SODIUM (MG)	CHOLESTEROL (MG)
Fats and oils	Nutiva Coconut Oil	1 tbsp (15 ml)	14	0	0	0	0	0
	Trader Joe's 100% Greek Kalamata Olive Oil	1 tbsp (15 ml)	14	0	0	0	0	0
Frozen	Trader Joe's Frozen Blueberries	¾ cup (74 g)	1	1	17	4	0	0
	Trader Joe's Pitted Dark Sweet Cherries	5 oz (141 g)	0	1	22	3	0	0
	Trader Joe's Wild Blackberries	1 cup (100 g)	0	1	17	4	0	0
Nuts and seeds	Fairway brand chia seeds	1 tbsp (10 g)	5	3	7	6	45	0
	Hampton Farms Unsalted Roasted Peanuts	1 oz (28 g) (shelled)	13	7	6	3	0	0
	Trader Joe's Almonds	½ cup (85 g)	15	6	7	4	0	0
	Trader Joe's Chia Seeds	1 tbsp (10 g)	5	3	7	6	0	0
	Trader Joe's Macadamias	¼ cup (38 g)	23	2	4	2	0	0
	Trader Joe's Pumpkin Seeds	¼ cup (31 g) (in shell)	13	9	4	2	75	0
	Trader Joe's Raw Shelled Hemp Seed	3 tbsp (30 g)	14	10	2	2	0	0
	Truck Roasted Hazelnuts	1 oz (28 g)	17	4	5	3	0	0
	Whole Foods bulk flaxseeds	2 tbsp (20 g)	8	4	7	6	5	0
	Whole Foods bulk raw pumpkin seeds	¼ cup (31 g)	14	9	4	3	5	0
	Whole Foods bulk sesame seeds	3 tbsp (30 g)	14	5	7	3	0	0
	Whole Foods Chia Powder	1 oz (28 g)	3	3	5	4	0	0
	Whole Foods Fresh Grind Almond Butter	¼ cup (45 g)	15	7	5	3	2	0
	Whole Foods Fresh Grind Peanut Butter	¼ cup (45 g)	18	9	8	3	0	0
	Whole Foods Fresh Grind Sprouted Almond Butter	¼ cup (45 g)	14	6	6	3	0	0
	Wonderful Pistachios	¼ cup (38 g)	14	6	8	3	160	0
	Wonderful Sweet Chili Pistachios	½ cup (76 g) with shells	14	6	8	3	290	0
Other	Nutiva Coconut Flour	2 tbsp (12 g)	2	4	11	8	20	0
	Red Mill Flaxseed Meal	2 tbsp (22 g)	4.5	3	4	4	0	0
	Red Mill Natural Almond Meal	¼ cup (24 g)	11	7	6	3	0	0
	Whole Foods bulk nutritional yeast	3 tbsp (28 g)	1	8	5	4	5	0

CATEGORY	FOOD ITEM	SERVING SIZE	FAT (G)	PROTEIN (G)	CARBS (G)	FIBER (G)	SODIUM (MG)	CHOLESTEROL (MG)
Pasta and pasta sauce	Amy's Family Marinara Pasta Sauce Light in Sodium	½ cup (125 g)	4.5	2	9	2	290	0
	Ancient Harvest Bean and Quinoa Pasta	2 oz (56 g)	1	12	35	7	0	0
	Ancient Harvest Lentil and Quinoa Pasta	2 oz (56 g)	1	14	35	7	0	0
	Cucina Antica tomato basil pasta sauce	½ cup (125 g)	1.5	1	6	2	240	0
Protein powders	Garden of Life Smooth Chocolate Plant Protein	1 scoop	2.5	15	6	3	180	0
	Garden of Life Smooth Energy Plant Protein	1 scoop	2	15	4	2	150	0
	Manitoba Forest Fiber Hemp Protein	4 tbsp (24 g)	4	11	14	13	0	0
	Nutiva Hi Fiber Hemp Protein	3 tbsp (18 g)	4	11	12	12	0	0
Snacks	Dr. Kracker Artisan Baked Crackers	6	5	6	13	4	220	0
	Eden Foods Dry Roasted Pumpkin Seeds	¼ cup (31 g)	16	10	5	5	100	0
	Eden Foods Quiet Moon Snacks	3 tbsp (38 g)	11	5	10	4	15	0
	Eden Foods Wild Berry Mix	3 tbsp (38 g)	8	5	13	4	10	0
	Go Raw Ginger Snaps	18 pieces	9	2	18	4	10	0
	Love Beets Organic Cooked Beets	¾ cup (134 g)	0	1	10	2	84	0
	Navitas Naturals Cacao Goji Power Snacks	1 oz (28 g)	5.9	3	15	2.5	50	0
	Red Mill Flaked Coconut	¼ cup (18 g)	10	1	4	2	5	0
	Righteously Raw Goji Cacao Bar	⅓ bar	7	1	9	2	20	0
	The Chia Company Chia Pod Vanilla Bean and Cinnamon	6 oz (170 g)	10	3	16	5	4	0
	The Good Bean Cracked Pepper Roasted Chickpeas	1 oz (28 g)	3	5	18	5	185	0
	The Good Bean Sea Salt Chickpeas	1 oz (28 g)	3	5	18	5	185	0
	Trader Joe's Roasted Seaweed Snack	½ package	2	1	1	1	50	0
	Trader Joe's Seasoned Kale Chips	½ package	7	4	12	2	180	0
	Trader Joe's Shelled Edamame	½ cup (76 g)	5	13	10	5	5	0
	Trader Joe's Triangulated Wasabi Trek Mix	¼ cup (50 g)	13	6	7	3	150	0
	Trader Joe's Wasabi Seaweed Snack	½ package	2	1	1	1	60	0
	Trader Joe's Zesty Nacho Kale Chips	1 oz (28 g)	9	6	11	3	220	0
	Whole Foods Golden Andan Berries	1 oz (28 g)	0	2	17	6	0	0
	Wild Garden Hummus Dip (All Flavors)	2 tbsp (28 g)	2	2	4	1	70	0

(continued)

CATEGORY	FOOD ITEM	SERVING SIZE	FAT (G)	PROTEIN (G)	CARBS (G)	FIBER (G)	SODIUM (MG)	CHOLESTEROL (MG)
Soups	Amy's Organic Lentil Soup Light in Sodium	1 cup (237 ml)	5	8	25	6	290	0
	Amy's Organic Low-Fat Minestrone Soup Light in Sodium	1 cup (237 ml)	1.5	3	17	3	290	0
	Bob's Red Mill Vegi Soup Mix	¼ cup (24 g) dry	1	11	36	13	0	0
	Pacific Low Sodium Vegetable Broth	1 cup (237 ml)	0	0	1	3	135	0
Vegetable protein	Hilary's Eat Well The World's Best Veggie Burger	1 piece	9	5	30	4	340	0
	Nasoya Tofu	3 oz (85 g)	4	8	2	1	5	0

Diabetic Resources

GENERAL REFERENCES

WebMD: http://www.webmd.com/diabetes/default.htm

Mayo Clinic: http://www.mayoclinic.org/diseases-conditions/diabetes/basics/definition/con-20033091

ADA: http://www.diabetes.org/

Joslin Diabetes Center: http://www.joslin.org/

The Genetic Landscape of Diabetes: http://www.ncbi.nlm.nih.gov/books/NBK1667/

CARBOHYDRATE COUNTING

Carbohydrate Counting: American Diabetes Association®: http://www.diabetes.org/food-and-fitness/food/what-can-i-eat/understanding-carbohydrates/carbohydrate-counting.html

Carbohydrate Counting 101: http://www.joslin.org/info/Carbohydrate_ Counting_101.html

Carbohydrate Counting and Diabetic Exchange Lists: http://fnic.nal.usda.gov/diet-and-disease/diabetes/carbohydrate-counting-and-exchange-lists

ACTIVITY TRACKERS

FitBit: www.fitbit.com/

Jawbone: https://jawbone.com/

Nike Fuel Band: http://www.nike.com/us/en_us/c/nikeplus-fuel

Microsoft Band: http://www.microsoft.com/microsoft-band/en-us

Apple Watch: https://www.apple.com/watch/

PLANT-BASED DIET GUIDELINES

Kaiser Permanente Plant-Based Diet Booklet: http://mydoctor.kaiserpermanente.org/ncal/Images/New%20Plant%20Based%20Booklet%201214_tcm28-781815.pdf

Plant-Based Diet for Beginners: http://www.mindbodygreen.com/0-952/PlantBased-Diet-for-Beginners-How-to-Get-Started.html

ACKNOWLEDGMENTS

This book would not have been possible without the hard work and support of the following:

Sharon Mahoney, the best adviser I could ever ask for; Sharon Bowers, my literary agent; Page Street Publishing; amazing recipe developer Jenny Dorsey; recipe tasters Irene Wu and Natalie Barbarese; and wonderful interns Elizabeth Canepari, Jessica Carciato and Bonnie Averbuch; all of my friends, colleagues and patients; and, of course, my family: my mom, my dad, my sister Liza, my grandmother and the rest of my incredible family.

Thank you!

ABOUT THE AUTHOR

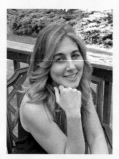 **Cher Pastore, MS, RDN, CDE,** is a registered dietitian and certified diabetes educator and the founder of CherNutrition, a private practice nutrition consulting business specializing in diabetes management. Passionate about guiding people to develop healthier lifestyles, Cher has spent the last 15 years providing nutrition consulting to doctors, clients and corporations on topics that include diabetes, weight management, prenatal and maternal nutrition, cardiovascular disease, digestive disorders, thyroid disorders and plant-based eating. Cher has spoken widely in the media about food and weight. She has been quoted in *Cosmopolitan, People* magazine *("The People Weight Loss Challenge")* and *Teen Vogue,* and has appeared on Fox News Channel's *Fox & Friends*, Channel 7 News and *Extra TV*. She lives and works in New York City and is a huge supporter of the JDRF and animal rights.

ENDNOTES

1   Key Findings. Report of the International Diabetes Federation, 2014, accessed January 31, 2015, http://www.idf.org/diabetesatlas/update-2014; "Off to the Right Start," International Diabetes Foundation, November 14, 2014, accessed January 31, 2015, http://www.idf.org/sites/default/files/wdd-press-kit-2014.pdf.

2   Ibid.

3   Ibid.

4   E. W. Gregg et al., "Trends in Lifetime Risk and Years of Life Lost Due to Diabetes in the USA, 1985–2011: A Modeling Study," *Lancet Diabetes Endocrinology 2 (2014): 867–74.*

5   Key Findings; "Off to the Right Start."

6   Ibid.

7   National Diabetes Statistics Report, Centers for Disease Control and Prevention, 2014, accessed September 8, 2014, http://www.cdc.gov/diabetes/pubs/statsreport14/national-diabetes-report-web.pdf.

8   Ibid.

9   "Standards of Medical Care in Diabetes: 2012," *Diabetes Care 35, supplement 1 (January 2012): S11–S63,* accessed September 14, 2014, http://care.diabetesjournals.org/content/35/Supplement_1/S11.full.pdf.

10   "Dietary Guidelines for Americans," US Department of Health and Human Services, n.d, accessed September 14, 2014, http://www.health.gov/dietaryguidelines/.

11   Scientific Report of the 2015 Dietary Guidelines Advisory Committee, Home of the Office of Disease Prevention and Health Promotion, February 2015.

12   http://www.cdc.gov/nchs/data/hestat/obesity_adult_11_12/obesity_adult_11_12.pdf

13   http://www.cdc.gov/nchs/data/hestat/obesity_child_11_12/obesity_child_11_12.pdf

14   National Diabetes Information Clearinghouse (NDIC), http://www.diabetes.niddk.nih.gov/.

15   "American Diabetes Association Releases New Research Estimating Annual Cost of Diabetes at $245 Billion," American Diabetes Association, March 6, 2013, accessed September 13, 2014, http://www.diabetes.org/newsroom/press-releases/2013/annual-costs-of-diabetes-2013.html.

16   "Prediabetes," Centers for Disease Control and Prevention, July 28, 2014, accessed September 5, 2014. http://www.cdc.gov/diabetes/consumer/prediabetes.htm.

17   National Diabetes Statistics Report.

18   Carlos A. Monteiro, "Nutrition and Health. The Issue Is Not Food, nor Nutrients, so Much as Processing," *Public Health Nutrition* 12, no. 5 (2009): 729.

19   Sheri R. Colberg, "Exercise and Type 2 Diabetes," *Diabetes Care* 33, no. 12 (2010), http://care.diabetesjournals.org/content/33/12/e147.abstract.

20   "Diagnosis and Classification of Diabetes," *Diabetes Care* 33, supplement 1 (2010), http://care.diabetesjournals.org/content/33/Supplement_1/S62.full.pdf html.

21   Joel Forman and Janet Silverstein, "Organic Foods: Health and Environmental Advantages and Disadvantages," *Pediatrics* 130, no. 5 (2012): 1406–15.

22   Adela Hruby, PhD, MPH, et al., "Higher Magnesium Intake Reduces Risk of Impaired Glucose and Insulin Metabolism, and Progression from Prediabetes to Diabetes in Middle-aged Americans," *Diabetes Care (October 2, 2013.*

23   R. A. DeFronzo and A. M. Goodman, "Efficacy of Metformin in Patients with Non-insulin-dependent Diabetes Mellitus," *New England Journal of Medicine 333 (1995: 541–49.)*

24   H. Khan, et al., "Vitamin D, Type 2 Diabetes and Other Metabolic Outcomes: A Systematic Review and Meta-analysis of Prospective Studies," *Proceedings of the Nutrition Society (2012).*

25   Richa Saxena, "Genome-wide Association Analysis Identifies Loci for Type 2 Diabetes and Triglyceride Levels," *Science 316, no. 5829 (2007): 1331–36.*

26   Patcharaporn Sudchada et al., "Effect of Folic Acid Supplementation on Plasma Total Homocysteine Levels and Glycemic Control in Patients with Type 2 Diabetes: A Systematic Review and Meta-analysis," *Diabetes Research and Clinical Practice* 98 (2012): 151–58.

INDEX